RHEUMATOLOGY EXAMINATION AND INJECTION TECHNIQUES

RHEUMATOLOGY EXAMINATION AND INJECTION TECHNIQUES

Michael Doherty

Consultant Senior Lecturer, Rheumatology Unit, City Hospital, Nottingham, UK

Brian L Hazleman

Consultant Rheumatologist, Rheumatology Research Unit, Addenbrooke's Hospital, Cambridge, UK

Charles W Hutton

Consultant Rheumatologist, Mount Gould Hospital, Plymouth, UK

Peter J Maddison

Professor of Bone and Joint Medicine, Royal National Hospital for Rheumatic Diseases, Upper Borough Walls, Bath, UK

J David Perry

Consultant Rheumatologist, The Royal London Hospital, Whitechapel, London, UK

W.B. Saunders Company Ltd

London   Philadelphia   Toronto   Sydney   Tokyo

W.B. Saunders Company Ltd

24–28 Oval Road
London NW1 7DX, UK

The Curtis Center
Independence Square West
Philadelphia, PA 19106–3399, USA

55 Horner Avenue
Toronto, Ontario M8Z 4X6, Canada

Harcourt Brace Jovanovich (Australia) Pty Ltd,
30–52 Smidmore St
Marrickville, NSW 2204, Australia

Harcourt Brace Jovanovich Japan Inc.
Ichibancho Central Building, 22–1 Ichibancho
Chiyoda-ku, Tokyo 102, Japan

© 1992 W.B. Saunders Company Ltd

This book is printed on acid free paper.

A catalogue record for this book is available from the British
Library.

ISBN 0–7020–1442–7

Typeset by Phoenix Photosetting, Chatham, Kent
Printed and bound in Great Britain by
Butler and Tanner Ltd, Frome, Somerset

CONTENTS

Colour plate section appears between p. 120 and p. 121

PREFACE

Rheumatological problems are exceedingly common in the community, may relate to disease in other systems, and are the single most important factor influencing disability in later life. The diagnosis and assessment of arthritis and periarticular lesions is almost entirely dependent on clinical skills and applied knowledge of regional anatomy. Unfortunately such skills are often poorly taught during student and specialist training in Europe and America, and many doctors feel less than competent in approaching examination of this large system.

This book represents the first combined approach to this topic by UK rheumatologists. It provides an introduction to important principles of the locomotor history and examination, proposes a brief screening procedure for regional localisation of problems, and then covers examination of each region in detail. Throughout, the emphasis is on common periarticular as well as articular abnormalities. Joint aspiration and periarticular/articular injection are common requirements for rheumatological assessment and management, and instruction on these techniques is, therefore, included for each region.

This book is particularly suited to trainees in rheumatology, but is also appropriate for trainee orthopaedic surgeons, general practice trainees and trainers, and interested allied health professionals. In addition the book contains enough detail to be of interest to established consultant rheumatologists.

Michael Doherty
Brian L Hazleman
Charles W Hutton
Peter J Maddison
J David Perry

INTRODUCTION TO EXAMINATION

I

INTRODUCTION

As its name suggests the locomotor system is primarily concerned with movement. The structure of its component tissues reflects this functional requirement, being designed to permit smooth efficient motion between articulating structures, while at the same time restraining and controlling excessive potentially harmful movement.

Development and Basic Structure of Joints

Bone, cartilage and muscle develop from mesenchymal tissue. Their basic structural features are self-differentiating, the chief aspects of differentiation occurring during the embryonic period (4th to 8th weeks). Mesenchymal tissues around the notochord segment to form primitive vertebrae from which dorsal and lateral projections subsequently form the neural arch and costal processes: occipital segments fuse to form part of the skull, and sacral segments fuse to form part of the pelvis. Limb buds appear in the cervical and lumbar segments and then grow peripherally, the proximal girdles migrating caudally but retaining their cervical nerve connections. By the end of the 8th week the embryo has assumed a recognisable human form, and the remainder of gestation (fetal period) is largely concerned with growth. During this period, and throughout subsequent life, locomotor development is strongly influenced by physical stresses associated with movement. Movement itself is thus one of the controlling forces that adapts the structure and organisation of locomotor tissues. Points worthy of note (particularly in respect of congenital skeletal anomalies) include:

- axial development occurs in a craniad–caudad manner.
- limb buds grow peripherally.

- upper limbs develop a little in advance of lower limbs (insults during the period of limb development affect a more distal portion of the upper extremity than of the lower extremity).
- the number of rays increases distally (one in upper arm and thigh, two in forearm and shin, three in carpus and tarsus, five in hand and foot).

Joints are discontinuities in the skeleton that permit controlled mobility. Their varying structure reflects varying functional requirements. If very little movement is required the bone-ends are firmly joined together in a continuous fashion (*synarthrosis*, Fig. 1). The two bones may be bridged by either:

- **Fibrous tissue** (*syndesmosis*), permitting almost no motion (e.g. skull sutures, interosseous membrane between radius and ulna), or
- **Cartilage** (*synchondrosis*), usually permitting a limited degree of movement. *Primary* cartilaginous joints, e.g. between epiphysis and diaphysis, are linked by hyaline cartilage which eventually ossifies. *Secondary* cartilaginous joints (*symphyses*) are joined by compressible fibrocartilage and reinforced by a surrounding tough fibrous capsule: they are predominantly axial (e.g. symphysis pubis, intervertebral joints, manubriosternal joints).

If a moderate or wide range of movement is required, a space must exist between the bones forming a discontinuous *diarthrosis* or *synovial joint* (Fig. 2). In synovial joints the bone ends are covered by hyaline cartilage, a firm but mildly compressible tissue ideally suited to load transmission. In some cases additional fibrocartilage pads divide the articular cavity completely (*discs*) or partially (*menisci*). An encircling *capsule* attaches between the bones: its outer portion is fibrous, its

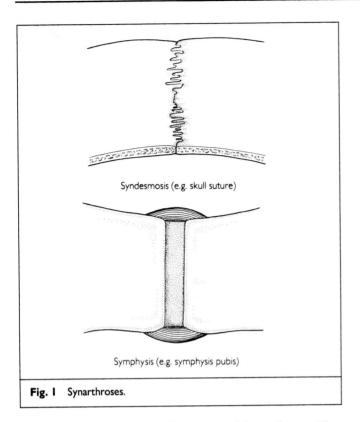

Syndesmosis (e.g. skull suture)

Symphysis (e.g. symphysis pubis)

Fig. I   Synarthroses.

inner lining forms the villous *synovial membrane*. The latter has both secretory and macrophage functions. It produces the viscous modified ultrafiltrate—*synovial fluid*—that fills the potential 'joint space', being important in lubrication and nutrition of cartilage. In many joints the synovium has multiple inward facing processes containing fat (*plicae*). *Ligaments* insert between the bones as thickened portions of capsule or as separate structures. The site of firm attachment of fibrous structures (tendon, ligament, capsule) into periosteum and bone is called the *enthesis*, a site frequently

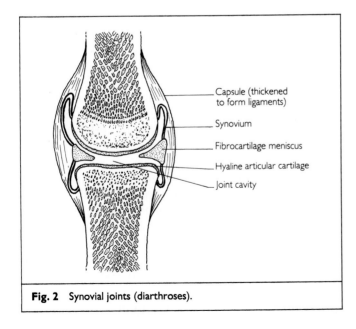

Capsule (thickened to form ligaments)

Synovium

Fibrocartilage meniscus

Hyaline articular cartilage

Joint cavity

Fig. 2   Synovial joints (diarthroses).

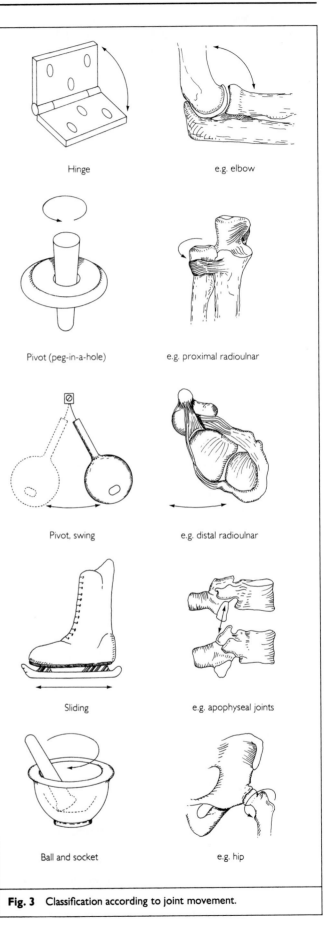

Hinge

e.g. elbow

Pivot (peg-in-a-hole)

e.g. proximal radioulnar

Pivot, swing

e.g. distal radioulnar

Sliding

e.g. apophyseal joints

Ball and socket

e.g. hip

Fig. 3   Classification according to joint movement.

inflamed through mechanical trauma or by involvement by inflammatory disease (particularly seronegative spondarthropathies).

Bursae are important fluid filled sacs which facilitate smooth movement between articulating structures. Their lining lacks a basement membrane and appears identical to synovium.

- **Subcutaneous bursae** (e.g. olecranon, prepatellar bursae) form only after birth in response to normal external friction.
- **Deep bursae** (e.g. subacromial bursa) usually form before birth in response to movement between muscles and bones, and may or may not communicate with adjacent joint cavities.
- **'Adventitious' bursae** (e.g. over 1st metatarsal head) form in response to abnormal shearing stresses and are not uniformly present.

Muscles acting over the joint move it through its normal range. Forceful movement in one direction is always controlled by relaxation of the antagonist muscles: the balanced action of muscles thus constrains as well as powers joint movement.

Tendons act as functional and anatomical bridges between muscle and bone. Muscle is unnecessary for the early differentiation of tendon, but without good muscle strength sustained development of tendon fails. Many tendons, particularly those with a wide range of motion, have sheaths resembling the capsule/synovium of joints to permit easy gliding movement.

The range of movement and stability of individual synovial joints varies according to:

- the shape of the articular surfaces,
- capsular strength,
- ligaments,
- muscles acting across the joint,
- the presence of adjacent structures.

Descriptive classification, especially of diarthrodial joints, is often based on the type of movement undertaken by the joint (Fig. 3).

Principles of the Rheumatological Examination

The rheumatological examination is very much an exercise in applied anatomy, with utilisation of simple provocation or stress tests to elicit signs. It cannot be over-emphasised that examination of the locomotor system should form an integral part of the full general medical examination. Many rheumatic diseases have manifestations in other systems and conversely many 'general medical' conditions (particularly endocrine, metabolic and neoplastic) have locomotor mani-

festations. In this introductory section, only locomotor history and examination will be considered: an accompanying full systems enquiry and examination is assumed, and aspects relating only to key target sites of extralocomotor involvement will be emphasised.

Terminology

The following brief glossary relates to terms commonly used to describe the site and nature of locomotor problems:

Arthralgia. Pain arising in joints (not necessarily with obvious abnormality).
Arthritis/Arthropathy. Objective joint abnormality.
Bursitis. Inflammation of a bursa.
Enthesopathy. Inflammation/abnormality of an enthesis.
Monoarthritis. Arthropathy of one joint only.
Myopathy. Disease/abnormality of muscle.
Myositis. Inflammatory disease of muscle.
Oligoarthritis/pauci-articular disease. Arthritis affecting two to four joints (or small joint groups, e.g. 'wrist').
Polyarthritis. Arthritis affecting more than four joints (or groups).
Synovitis. Clinically apparent synovial joint inflammation.
Tenosynovitis. Tendon sheath inflammation.
Tendinitis. Inflammation of tendon.

Symptoms

Locomotor symptoms requiring clear delineation in the history are summarised in Figure 4. It is important to ascertain:

- the site and distribution of involvement,
- chronological onset,

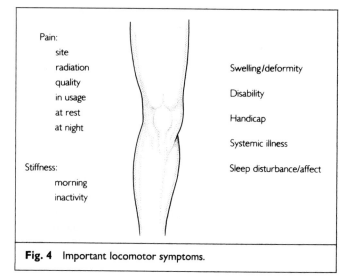

Fig. 4 Important locomotor symptoms.

- preceding provoking factors,
- factors which worsen or improve symptoms,
- symptom response to health interventions.

Pain

Pain is the usual and most important symptom for which the patient seeks relief. The examiner must be in no doubt as to where the patient is experiencing pain. Patient vocabulary alone (e.g. 'shoulder', 'hip') may be misleading and the patients should be asked to point to and delineate on their own body the area over which they feel pain and the site of maximum intensity.

Articular or periarticular pain may radiate widely and present distant from the originating structure (Fig. 5). Such pain felt elsewhere than at its origin is termed *referred*. Referred pain is an error in perception at the sensory cortex level, reflecting shared innervation from structures derived from the same embryonic segment (which divides into dermatome, myotome, sclerotome). Sensory (including painful) stimuli reaching cortical cells will most commonly originate from a certain area of skin: when the same cells receive for the first time a painful stimulus from a more deep-seated structure (myotomal or sclerotomal origin) they interpret the signal on past experience and 'feel' the pain in the area of skin (dermatome) connected with those particular cortical cells. An important difference, however, is that the pain is felt deeply rather than in the skin itself. Certain joints are relevant to such referred pain:

- Pain radiates segmentally without crossing the midline.
- The extent of the relevant dermatome governs the distance pain may radiate. Extensive referral only occurs where elongated segments exist (i.e. limbs).
- The dermatome often extends more distally than the myotome, so pain is usually referred predominantly in a distal direction. The more distal the originating structure the more accurate the pain localisation is likely to be.
- Dermatomes are extremely variable between individuals—subsequently the precise pattern and area of pain referral may vary between individuals with the same originating musculoskeletal problem.
- In general, the more superficial a soft-tissue structure the more precise its localising ability. Pain is apt to be referred from capsule, ligament, muscle and bursa in an indistinguishable manner. Pain from bone and periosteum, however, hardly radiates at all, and this discrepancy between soft and hard structures is unexplained.

Detailed questioning on the descriptive *quality* of pain is generally unhelpful. Exceptions, however, include (1) sharp shooting pain that travels a distance, characteristic of root entrapment, and (2) extreme pain ('worst experienced'), which is typical of crystal synovitis. Although topographical localisation of sensation is at the sensory cortex level, the fact that it is painful and the degree of pain experienced is determined by cells in the supraorbital region of the frontal lobes. Such localisation explains why the patient's emotional state has such a profound influence over pain 'severity'. The temporal lobes retain the memory of pain, and it is the duration rather than the severity which principally determines recollection.

Factors which exacerbate or ameliorate the pain should obviously be sought. It is convenient to consider locomotor pain in terms of *usage*, *rest* and *night* pain. Pain confined to *usage* suggests a mechanical problem, particularly if it worsens during use and quickly improves on resting. *Rest pain* and pain worse at the beginning rather than end of usage implies a pronounced inflammatory component. *Night pain* is a distressing symptom that often carries a poor prognosis: it predominently associates with marked intraosseous hypertension and may therefore denote serious problems such as avascular necrosis or subchondral bone collapse adjacent to a severely arthritic joint. Persistent day and night pain is particularly worrying, and such *bony pain* is characteristic of neoplastic invasion.

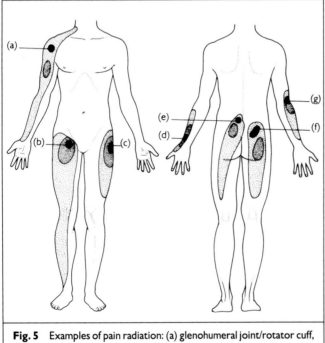

Fig. 5 Examples of pain radiation: (a) glenohumeral joint/rotator cuff, (b) hip joint, (c) trochanteric bursitis, (d) de Quervain's tenosynovitis, (e) lumbar facet joint syndrome, (f) sacroiliac joint, (g) tennis elbow syndrome.

Stiffness

Stiffness is a sensation of tightness that can usually 'wear off'. In simplistic terms it can be thought of as fluid accumulation that distends the limiting boundary of the inflamed tissue (e.g. joint capsule, tenosynovium, bursa). It is most marked on (1) first arising in the morning (following relative inactivity during sleep), and (2) following inactivity or rest of the inflamed region. As the region resumes the movement of normal usage, fluid clearance from the inflamed structure is encouraged and stiffness 'wears off'. Duration and severity of *early morning* and *inactivity stiffness* are therefore important indicators of the degree of local inflammation.

Swelling/deformity

Patients themselves may notice swelling (which could be soft tissue, fluid or bone), discoloration or an abnormal contour or alignment of a locomotor structure. Strictly speaking, 'deformity' is anything out of the ordinary; the term is usually reserved, however, for a malalignment or subluxation/dislocation (the latter terms, rather than deformity, are preferable during discussions with the patient).

Disability and handicap

Disability is present when a tissue, organ or system is unable to adequately perform its function. Such disability may lead to *handicap* if it interferes with daily activities or social/occupational performance. Marked disability need not necessarily cause handicap (e.g. an above-knee amputee may not be disadvantaged in a sedentary job); similarly, minor disability may produce major handicap (e.g. a bunion in a professional athlete). The two must therefore be assessed separately, the history being particularly important in determining handicap.

Systemic illness

Inflammatory locomotor disease, particularly with multisystem involvement, may trigger a marked acute phase response and lead to symptoms of systemic upset. Patients may notice low-grade fevers (particularly at night), weight loss, fatiguability, lethargy, and irritability. Often the patient volunteers no specific complaints but just feels generally 'ill' ('malaise'). In the elderly particularly, florid inflammation (e.g. acute gout or pseudogout) may cause toxic confusion.

Sleep disturbance/affect

There may be several reasons for poor sleep in patients with locomotor disease:

- Any chronic painful condition may interfere with sleep (such interruption may play a part in the fibromyalgia syndrome).

- Triggering of the acute phase response may affect normal sleep patterns.
- Severe arthropathy (particularly hip and knee) may compromise sexual function, and contribute to marital/social disharmony.
- Latent anxiety and depression is not uncommon in patients with severe arthropathy, perhaps resulting from reasonable concern about deformity, function and morbidity.
- Some drugs used for pain relief (e.g. indomethacin) may produce CNS side-effects with alteration in sleep and mood.

Features of masked or overt depression (e.g. psychomotor retardation, constipation, weepiness, no thoughts of the future) should specifically be sought, particularly in those with severe locomotor problems. Poor sleep pattern is also a feature of fibromyalgia.

Signs

The principal headings for signs to be sought at any region are shown in Figure 6. The order of examination applicable to most regions is:

1. inspection at rest,
2. inspection during movement,
3. palpation.

Attitude

The way in which the patient positions an affected region or limb may provide important clues to the underlying problem. Any inflamed joint with synovitis has intra-articular hypertension and is most comfortable in the position that minimises pressure increase. The position of maximum comfort is mainly determined by the capsule and the ligamentous

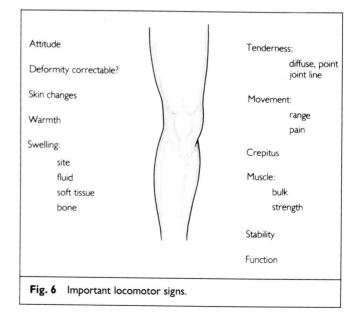

Attitude

Deformity correctable?

Skin changes

Warmth

Swelling:
    site
    fluid
    soft tissue
    bone

Tenderness:
    diffuse, point
    joint line

Movement:
    range
    pain

Crepitus

Muscle:
    bulk
    strength

Stability

Function

Fig. 6 Important locomotor signs.

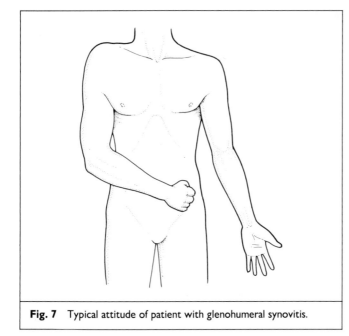

Fig. 7 Typical attitude of patient with glenohumeral synovitis.

Table 1. Causes of erythema overlying joints

MAJOR
sepsis
crystals (gout, pseudogout, calcific periarthritis)

MINOR
palindromic rheumatism
acute Reiter's syndrome, reactive arthropathy
erythema nodosum
early Heberden's and Bouchard's nodes
inflammatory ('erosive') osteoarthritis of hands
rheumatic fever

Erythema implies associated periarticular inflammation

arrangement: the position is that of greatest laxity which allows maximum intracapsular capacity. In general this is a position of mild–mid flexion (i.e. the fetal position). For example, a patient with gleno-humeral synovitis (Fig. 7) is most comfortable if the arm is held in adduction and internal rotation (as if in a sling): equally, the earliest affected and most uncomfortable movements are the opposite of these, namely abduction and external rotation, since these maximally increase intra-articular pressure. The attitude and pattern of restricted movement may thus suggest the diagnosis.

Deformity
Although deformities may readily be observed at rest, many will become more apparent on weight bearing or

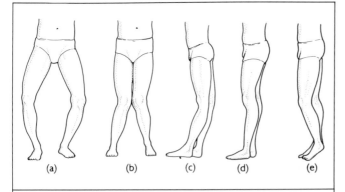

Fig. 8 Principal knee deformities. (a) *Varus:* typical of osteoarthritis (a focal condition maximally affecting the medial compartment). (b) *Valgus:* typical of pancompartment inflammatory conditions, e.g. rheumatoid, psoriatic, pyrophosphate arthropathy. (c) *Recurvatum:* common in generalised hypermobility. (d) *Posterior tibial subluxation:* characteristic of arthritis occurring during growth, e.g. haemophilia. (e) *Fixed flexion:* common in various arthropathies.

usage. It should be determined whether the deformity is *correctable* (usually implying soft tissue factors in causation) or *non-correctable* (more commonly capsular restriction, joint damage). Many conditions associate with characteristic deformities (e.g. at the knee, Fig. 8), but no deformity is pathognomonic of any one disease. Shorthand terms are often used for combined deformities (e.g. 'swan neck' deformity for hyperextension at the proximal and hyperflexion at the distal interphalangeal joints of the same finger).

Skin changes
Overlying traumatic/surgical scars or skin disease (e.g. psoriasis) may be important clues to causation. *Erythema* (commonly followed by desquamation) is an important sign that reflects periarticular inflammation. Although this may occur in several conditions (Table 1), a red joint (or bursa) should always raise suspicion of sepsis or crystals.

Warmth
This is one of the cardinal signs of inflammation and should be sought over bursae, tendon sheaths, entheses and joints (non-axial joints that are not deep in soft tissues are readily accessible for temperature assessment). The back of the hand is a sensitive thermometer for comparing skin temperature above, over and below an inflamed structure.

Swelling
This may be due to *fluid, soft tissue* or *bone*. Fluid within a joint collects initially and maximally at sites of least resistance within the capsular confines, producing a characteristic swelling at individual joint sites, for example:

• *A knee effusion* initially fills in the medial dimple at the side of the patella and subsequently the suprapatellar pouch, giving a horseshoe swelling above and to either side of the patella (Fig. 9).

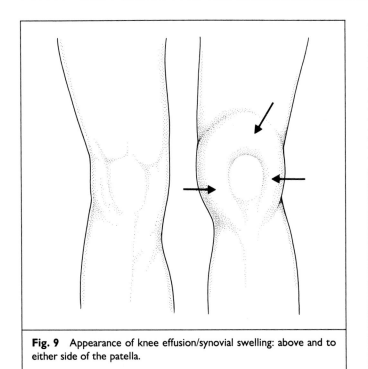

Fig. 9 Appearance of knee effusion/synovial swelling: above and to either side of the patella.

- *Interphalangeal joint synovitis* is initially apparent as posterolateral swelling between the extensor tendon and lateral collateral ligaments (Fig. 10).
- *Glenohumeral effusion* initially fills the triangular depression between clavicle and deltoid in front of pectoralis.
- *Ankle effusions* present anteriorly.

For fluid within an anatomically confined space

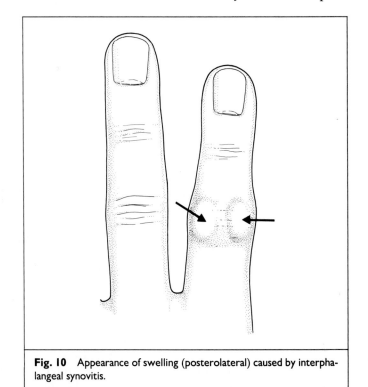

Fig. 10 Appearance of swelling (posterolateral) caused by interphalangeal synovitis.

several signs may be elicited. A small fluid volume may produce a *bulge sign* if it is gently massaged from one side of the space to the other (readily demonstrable at the knee by flicking fluid from the medial dimple to the lateral aspect of the patella and back again; Fig. 11). A larger volume abolishes the bulge sign but permits elucidation of a *balloon sign* where pressure exerted at one point of the swelling is felt as 'ballooning' at other parts of the swelling (Fig. 12). This is

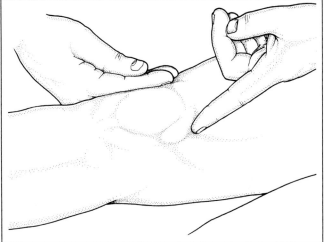
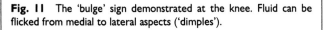

Fig. 11 The 'bulge' sign demonstrated at the knee. Fluid can be flicked from medial to lateral aspects ('dimples').

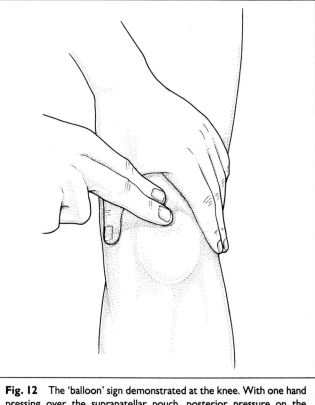

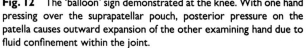

Fig. 12 The 'balloon' sign demonstrated at the knee. With one hand pressing over the suprapatellar pouch, posterior pressure on the patella causes outward expansion of the other examining hand due to fluid confinement within the joint.

the most specific sign for fluid in joints or bursae. *Capsular swelling* is the most specific sign of synovitis: swelling is delineated by the capsular confines and becomes firmer as the joint moves towards the extremes of movement (palpate during passive movement).

Tenderness

Precise localisation of tenderness is perhaps the most useful sign in determining the cause of the patient's problem.

Joint-line/capsular tenderness is localised to the joint boundary and signifies arthropathy or capsular disease if present around the whole joint margin. Localised, rather than generalised, joint-line tenderness may reflect problems with an intracapsular structure (e.g. anterior medial tibiofemoral compartment tenderness at the knee is common with medial meniscal tears).

Periarticular point tenderness away from the joint line usually signifies bursitis or enthesopathy.

Movement

The range of both *active* and *passive* movement can readily be assessed with comparison of one side to the other. Synovitis usually reduces most or all joint movements (though some are effected initially and maximally, e.g. external rotation and abduction at the glenohumeral joint). Each joint has a characteristic pattern of such *'proportional'* limitation (*'capsular pattern'*), governed largely by the capsular and ligamentous arrangement that determines intracapsular pressure changes on movement. Tenosynovitis and periarticular lesions more commonly affect movement in one plane only (i.e. the plane of movement of the involved structure). Such a *'non-capsular'* pattern of restriction may also result from an internal derangement (only certain joints such as the knee and elbow are affected in this way). Synovitis and arthropathy usually result in similar reduction of both active and passive movement: passive movement far greater than active movement suggests a muscle/tendon/motor problem.

The pattern of pain elicited by movement is of great diagnostic significance. Pain absent or minimal in the mid-range position but increasing progressively towards the extremes of restricted movement is *stress pain* (Fig. 13). *Universal stress pain* (i.e. in most/all directions) is the most sensitive sign of synovitis (Table 2). *Selective stress pain* (i.e. in one plane of movement only) is characteristic of a localised lesion in or around a joint. Pain uniformly present throughout a range of movement usually reflects mechanical rather than inflammatory problems.

Ranges of joint movement are age-, sex- and race-dependent, and are difficult to quantify with any

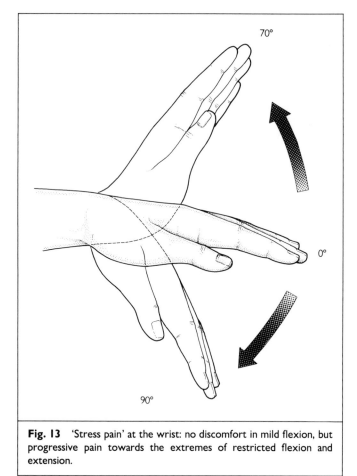

Fig. 13 'Stress pain' at the wrist: no discomfort in mild flexion, but progressive pain towards the extremes of restricted flexion and extension.

accuracy (other than by radiographic techniques). Direct comparison of one side with the other may be helpful in demonstrating unilateral reduction. Attempts to measure degrees of movement (by a variety of instruments) are inaccurate, have poor reproducibility and are not recommended.

A principle used at several sites for demonstrating muscle tendon or enthesis problems is *resisted active (isometric) movement* (Fig. 14). The patient is asked to push against the examiner's restraining hand, to contract the muscle of interest without moving adjacent joints (to minimise the chance of joint or surrounding inert tissue movement, the joint is placed in a neutral or resting position). If the patient's pain is reproduced by this manoeuvre (and no joint or surrounding inert tissue has moved) it is likely that the pain arises from the muscle, tendon or tendon insertion related to that movement. For example, resisted adduction at the hip may reproduce medial groin pain in adductor tendonitis; resisted glenohumeral abduction may produce upper arm pain with supraspinatus muscle or tendon lesions; and resisted active wrist extension may produce pain at the lateral epicondyle in tennis elbow. Similarly, *passive stress tests* may be applied in an attempt to reproduce the patient's pain by stretching the responsible ligament or tendon (e.g. Finkelstein's

Table 2. Characteristic findings in an inflamed joint (synovitis), tenosynovitis and a damaged joint

SYNOVITIS
Most comfortable in neutral position
Decreased movement *all* planes
Stress pain *all* directions
Capsular swelling/effusion
Joint-line/capsular tenderness
Warmth
± Fine crepitus

> *Capsular swelling = most specific sign*
> *Stress pain = most sensitive sign*

TENOSYNOVITIS
Joint positioned to decrease tension on tendon
Decreased movement in plane of tendon
Selective stress pain
Linear swelling
Localised (linear) tenderness
± Fine crepitus
± Triggering

JOINT DAMAGE
Abnormal shape
Coarse crepitus
Decreased movement
± Ligamentous stress pain/instability
± Synovitis

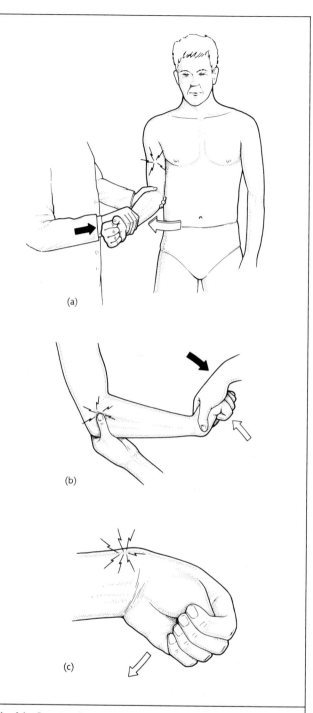

Fig. 14 Restricted active movement and stress tests: (a) Attempted external rotation at the shoulder causing upper arm pain in infraspinatus/teres minor rotator cuff lesion. (b) Resisted wrist extension reproducing lateral epicondyle pain in tennis elbow. (c) Finkelstein's test: passive ulnar flexion with the thumb held stretches abductor pollicis longus and extensor pollicis brevis to reproduce pain of de Quervain's tenosynovitis.

test for De Quervain's tenosynovitis, where passive stretch of abductor pollicis longus and extensor pollicis brevis reproduces pain).

Crepitus
Crepitus is palpable crunching present throughout the range of movement of the involved structure. *Fine crepitus* may be audible by stethoscope and is not transmitted through bone adjacent to the involved structure; it may accompany inflammation of tendon sheath, bursa or synovium. *Coarse crepitus* may be audible at a distance and is often palpable through adjacent bone: it usually reflects cartilage or bone damage. Other locomotor noises include *ligamentous snaps* (usually single, loud and painless: commonly heard around the greater trochanter region as 'clicking hips'); *cracking* by joint distraction (common at finger joints and caused by formation of an intra-articular gas bubble subsequent to the negative pressure generated: such painless and inconsequential 'cracking' cannot be repeated until the bubble has resorbed); and a variety of reproducible *clonking* noises at irregular surfaces (e.g. moving the scapula over the thoracic wall).

Muscle
Muscle wasting is a common but difficult sign, particularly in women and older patients in whom muscle contour is normally less striking. Synovitis will quickly produce reflex inhibition of muscles acting across the

Table 3. Muscle power grading (Medical Research Council scale)

Grade	Muscle power
0	No visible contraction
1	Visible or palpable contraction without motion
2	Motion only with gravity eliminated
3	Motion against gravity
4	Motion against gravity and an applied load
5	Normal, i.e. against a significant load

Table 4. Generalised hypermobility defined using a Carter and Wilkinson score (modified by Beighton)

Extend little finger >90° (1 point each)
Bring back thumb parallel to/touching forearm (1 point each)
Extend elbow >10° (1 point each)
Extend knee >10° (1 point each)
Touch floor with flat of hands, legs straight (1 point)

Maximum score = 9 (6+ = hypermobile)

joint by local spinal reflex: wasting of muscle can occur very quickly (e.g. within 2–3 days in septic arthritis). Severe arthropathy commonly produces widespread wasting of muscles around the joint: localised wasting is more characteristic of a mechanical tendon/muscle problem or peripheral nerve damage. Power is more important than bulk and should be tested, either by formal testing using MRC grades 0–5 (Table 3: appropriate, for example, for proximal girdle and neck muscle weakness in polymyositis) or by assessment of functional capabilities (suitable, for example, for weakness of small hand muscles in polyarticular rheumatoid).

Stability
Localised ligamentous or capsular instability may result from traumatic or inflammatory lesions: direct comparison with the other side (and with other joints) should always be made in case this represents part of generalised hypermobility. Inflammatory joint disease (particularly rheumatoid) may produce instability via cartilage loss and capsular inflammation, as well as by ligamentous rupture.

Function
Function for each joint region is assessed by observation during normal usage (e.g. rising from chair and walking, for assessing hips, knees and feet; power grip and fine precision pinch for assessing the hand). *Activities of daily living* (e.g. dressing, brushing teeth, turning handles, going to the toilet unaided, cooking) are of principal relevance to the patient, and screening questions or observations of such movements ('ADL') are invaluable in assessment. Handicap is mainly determined by questioning in respect of work and social activities. A number of tested and validated questionnaires/scoring systems are available for *functional* and *quality of life assessments*. The latter particularly depends on physical, psychological and emotional factors, which are highly specific to the patient rather than to the condition.

Two generalised conditions are easily missed unless specifically considered:

Generalised hypermobility. Approximately 10% of people fall within the lax end of a normal spectrum of joint mobility. Although normal, such hypermobility may contribute to locomotor problems (e.g. enthesopathy, dislocation). Within this 10% are also the small number of individuals with disease-related hypermobility (e.g. Marfan's syndrome, Ehlers–Danlos syndrome, acromegaly). Generalised hypermobility can be screened for using a modified Beighton score (Table 4).

Fibromyalgia (non-restorative sleep disorder). This common syndrome is characterised by:
- poor sleep pattern (waking unrefreshed),
- fatiguability, lethargy,
- irritability, weepiness,
- multiple regional pain problems (predominantly axial, often 'all over'), usually unresponsive to analgesics,
- hypersensitivity of normal tender sites (Fig. 15),
- frequent accompanying 'tension' headaches and irritable bowel syndrome.

Fibromyalgia may be *primary* (particularly affecting middle-aged women) or *secondary*, superimposed on a recognised locomotor or chronic painful condition ('pain amplification syndrome'). It is suggested by the features in the history and confirmed principally by the finding of hypertender sites (with no hyperalgesia at other, control sites) and elimination of other causes

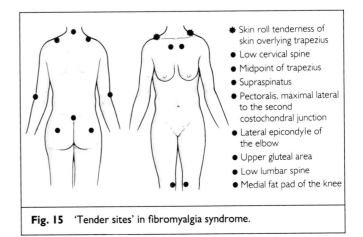

* Skin roll tenderness of skin overlying trapezius
• Low cervical spine
• Midpoint of trapezius
• Supraspinatus
• Pectoralis, maximal lateral to the second costochondral junction
• Lateral epicondyle of the elbow
• Upper gluteal area
• Low lumbar spine
• Medial fat pad of the knee

Fig. 15 'Tender sites' in fibromyalgia syndrome.

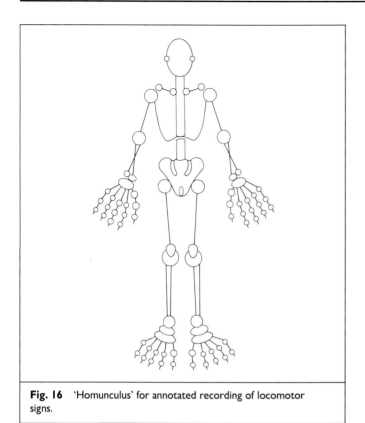

Fig. 16 'Homunculus' for annotated recording of locomotor signs.

Table 5. Causes of nodules and arthropathy

COMMON
Rheumatoid arthritis
Gout (= 'tophi')
Hyperlipidaemia (= 'xanthomata')

RARE
Systemic lupus erythematosus (small nodules)
Rheumatic fever
Polyarteritis nodosa
Multicentric reticulohistiocytosis
Sarcoidosis

alveolitis are particularly relevant); 'thimble pitting', onycholysis and nail dystrophy (psoriatic arthropathy, chronic Reiter's syndrome); and splinter haemorrhages (small vessel vasculitis). Rheumatoid arthritis is the commonest pathologic cause of *palmar erythema* (more so than cirrhosis and thyrotoxicosis; pregnancy is a common physiological cause).

Table 6. Important causes of a red eye

CONJUNCTIVITIS
Itchiness, irritation
Diffusely red due to engorged vessel network
Redness extends over bulbar surface of eyelids
Vessels can be moved over surface
Mucopurulent discharge common ('sticky eye')

EPISCLERITIS
Usually asymptomatic
Diffuse or localised ('nodular' episcleritis)
Bright red flush, individual vessels often visible
Vessels cannot be moved over eyeball
Vessels constrict to local adrenaline drops (1:1000)

SCLERITIS
Usually painful, often severe
Deep red/purple colour, vessels indistinct
Deep vessels do not constrict to adrenaline drops
Often accompanied by episcleritis
Localised ('nodular') scleritis causes elevated lesion due to oedema
Diffuse scleritis causes less pain but may involve cornea, causing keratitis and keratolysis ('corneal melt')
Healed scleritis may leave sclera more transparent and permit the dark underlying choroid to be seen

ACUTE IRITIS
Severe, throbbing pain
Blurring of vision, photophobia, lacrimation
Usually involves only one eye at a time: light in other eye will exacerbate pain as iris constricts
Small vessels of limbus are engorged ('ciliary flush')
Small spastic pupil, may be irregular (due to posterior adhesions or synechiae)
Clouding of aqueous ± anterior chamber pus collection inferiorly ('hypopyon')

of widespread aches and pains (e.g. hyperparathyroidism, hypothyroidism, lupus, etc.). Unless specifically considered it is easily missed.

Recording of locomotor signs

Although it is feasible to record physical findings in note form, annotation around skeleton charts or homunculi (Fig. 16) is strongly recommended. Such a visual method of recording greatly aids pattern recognition.

Aspects of the general examination

In the context of a complete systems examination particular emphasis may be given to skin (including scalp, umbilicus and natal cleft for occult psoriasis), nails, mucous membranes, and eyes. It cannot be overemphasised, however, that a full medical history and examination should be undertaken.

Nodules are a feature of particular relevance to locomotor disease (Table 5). Whatever the cause, they are usually most prominent over extensor surfaces with poor soft-tissue covering (e.g. back of hand, elbow, posterior heel, sacrum).

Nail changes of interest include clubbing (most causes of clubbing have locomotor associations, but hypertrophic pulmonary osteoarthropathy and fibrosing

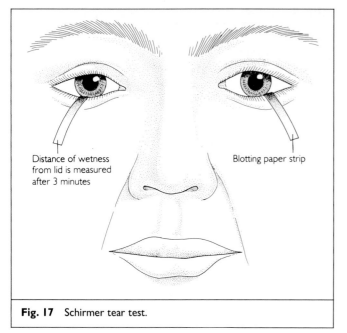

Fig. 17 Schirmer tear test.

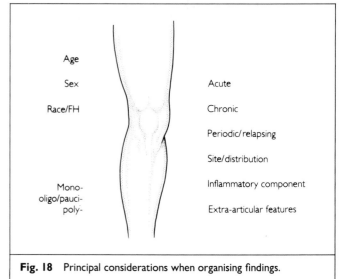

Fig. 18 Principal considerations when organising findings.

Mucous membrane lesions may be asymptomatic (Reiter's/reactive arthropathy) or symptomatic (usual in lupus, vasculitides, Behçet's syndrome), and inspection of orogenital and nasal mucosae for ulcers and telangiectasia is warranted. Absence of saliva either side of the frenulum suggests sicca syndrome (patients often complain of dry mouth, particularly in the morning, and difficulty swallowing certain foods: dry eyes are more commonly asymptomatic).

Eye changes (Table 6) include *episcleritis* and *scleritis* (rheumatoid arthritis, vasculitides, polychondritis); *iritis* (ankylosing spondylitis, chronic Reiter's syndrome); iridocyclitis (pauciarticular juvenile chronic arthritis); and *conjunctivitis* (acute Reiter's syndrome, sicca syndrome). A Schirmer tear test is a simple screen for sicca syndrome; although it may produce false positives and negatives, it may readily be performed without special equipment (Fig. 17). Confirmation of sicca syndrome is by Rose Bengal staining and slit-lamp examination (histological evidence is most commonly sought by lip biopsy to show minor salivary gland changes).

Assimilation of findings

Following the history and examination it is often helpful to organise findings under the titles in Figure 18.

Making a diagnosis rarely presents problems once the clinically derived information is collected and considered. Problems and misdiagnosis most commonly arise if an inadequate or inaccurate history and examination have failed to elicit the correct information in the first instance.

Consideration just of age and sex will narrow diagnostic possibilities considerably. Occasionally genetic factors (race, family history) may suggest or support a particular diagnosis, though a positive history (which may of course be inaccurate in terms of precise diagnosis in family members) is as often misleading as it is helpful, and most store should be placed on the individual patient findings. For arthropathy in a patient of a certain age and sex the temporal presentation (acute, chronic or relapsing), number of joints involved, distribution, and degree of inflammatory component (assessed from both symptoms and signs) will usually suggest the most likely diagnosis, with a few alternatives. The presence of particular extra-articular features may narrow possibilities further. Investigations, if required, can then be highly selected, and a rheumatological 'screen' with multiple investigations should never be necessary. It should be remembered, however, that apparently mundane and localised lesions (e.g. Achilles tendinitis) may be the presenting feature of a more widespread or multisystem condition.

Only an adequate history and examination will permit correct diagnosis and an appropriate management plan.

THE MINIMUM RHEUMATOLOGICAL EXAMINATION

In terms of physical examination the locomotor system is extensive and complex. An exhaustive history and examination for all conceivable rheumatological abnormalities in every patient would not only be very time-consuming but also inefficient and unnecessary. As with the neurological examination (and to a lesser extent other systems examination), a brief screening procedure to pick up problems in certain regions is more appropriate. If an abnormality is detected, more detailed examination of the affected region(s) (as described in subsequent chapters) can then be undertaken.

A screening procedure represents a compromise between brevity and reasonable sensitivity for detecting abnormality. Every physician must develop his or her own personal variation of the 'minimum survey' for the locomotor just as for other systems, and the procedure described in this section is offered as a guide rather than didactic doctrine. Such a survey, however, is reasonable to include as a 'minimal statement' within the systems enquiry and examination screen that comprises the routine medical clerking. Furthermore, such a survey should form a component of the basic examination that lies within the scope of all practising doctors and is performed so routinely as to become 'reflex' in nature. Certain aspects of the screen (e.g. gait) might be undertaken during screening of other systems and, in the context of a full examination, takes only an extra minute or so to perform.

Screening History

Pain and stiffness are the two most common symptoms relating to locomotor abnormality, and impairment of function is the most important common consequence. The following are therefore reasonable screening questions for rheumatological disease:

Have you any pain or stiffness in your muscles, joints or back?
Can you dress yourself completely without any difficulty?
Can you walk up and down stairs without any difficulty?

Dressing is a daily event and one with which the patient will readily identify in terms of problems. Ability to dress completely (including shoes and socks) is a sensitive functional test of most upper and lower limb joints, and if the patient has no pain or difficulty performing this task then significant or widespread locomotor disease is unlikely. If the patient can ascend and descend stairs without pain or difficulty then most lower limb muscles and joints (large and small) are functioning well: walking on the flat is also unlikely to present problems (up and down stairs is a better test of hip and knee, particularly patello-femoral, problems than walking on the flat). If none of these questions pick up a problem then further questioning is unlikely to do so. If a problem is detected, more detailed questioning should obviously be undertaken.

Screening Examination

The main emphasis is on inspection at rest and inspection during selected movements which are affected early by joint disease. Brief palpation and stress tests of target joint sites (e.g. metacarpophalangeal joints—MCPJs, metatarsophalangeal joints—MTPJs, knees) completes the screen.

If a joint is normal it should:

1. *Look normal.* With advancing age the surface contours of a joint become more visible, and muscle bulk diminishes, without necessarily having pathological significance.
2. *Assume a normal resting position.* Each joint has a characteristic resting position. Abnormal positioning of a normal joint may result from poor posture, neurological abnormality, or psychogenic disorder with feigning of disease. Postural abnormalities should disappear once the patient is asked to adopt the normal position and undertake normal movements.
3. *Move smoothly through its range of movement.* Articular or periarticular lesions often result in a jerky, guarded movement, and the patient may utilise trick manoeuvres to minimise any functional problem.

The order of screening is of little consequence. Each practitioner develops his or her own order and, with practice, inspection, palpation and stress tests of a region can often be undertaken at the same time. Description of the patient assessment is conveniently considered during three activities: during walking, while standing and while lying on a couch. Observation of the patient getting undressed is a further useful screen to detect functional problems in upper and lower limb joints (though some physicians prefer to spare the patient any embarrassment this may cause).

Inspection of the walking patient

With the patient barefoot and undressed to his or her underwear, observe the patient's gait over a minimum of several yards as he or she walks forwards, turns and walks back again. Carefully inspect movements of the arms, pelvis, hips, knees, hindfoot, midfoot and forefoot in turn. Normal gait (Fig. 1) is characterised by:

- easy, flowing movement of each arm linked with co-ordinated movement of the opposite leg;
- symmetrical movement of the pelvis, smoothly rotating forward with the advancing leg;
- flexion of the hip at heel-strike, extension at toe-off;
- knee extension at heel-strike, flexion during swing;
- normal heel-strike, foot pronation in mid-stance,

heel rise before push-off, and ankle dorsiflexion during swing;
- smooth turning ability.

As the patient walks and turns look particularly for an *antalgic gait*; where, pain or deformity causes the patient to hurry off one leg and to spend most of the gait cycle on the other. The type of antalgic gait may suggest the region that is abnormal. For example:

Low back problem. Decreased rotation of the pelvis with the advancing leg leads to a shortened step and caution when turning.

Hip problem. The body 'bobs' over the painful side: fixed flexion accentuates lumbar lordosis and exaggerates buttock prominence.

Knee problem. Synovitis/deformity may prevent full extension during swing and soften heel-strike. If the knee is ankylosed or held stiffly, the body pivots around the leg during stance phase and the leg is swung forward by circumduction.

Hindfoot problem. If movement through the ankle is reduced, the leg may be externally rotated and slightly abducted. With heel-pain, heel-strike may be replaced by 'foot-strike': the heel is kept off the floor and the knee does not fully extend. With Achilles tendon problems, push-off is avoided.

Mid-foot problem. The foot is held inverted (supinated) and push-off is from the lateral side.

Forefoot problem. To prevent weight-bearing on the forefoot the heel does not rise in late stance, and there is no push-off. The knee, hip and trunk flex to maintain forward motion, and swing phase on the normal side is shortened, resulting in forward 'bobbing' during late stance on the painful side. Involvement of both forefeet combines to give a forward leaning, short-stepped, shuffling gait.

Additional abnormalities include a *Trendelenburg gait* (the pelvis drops down on the opposite side during stance phase on the affected side—due to ineffective hip abduction), a *waddling gait* (i.e. a bilateral Trendelenburg gait), and *hysterical/psychogenic* gaits (often variable, exaggerated or bizarre, conforming to no easily recognised pattern).

If the observed gait is entirely normal, the patient is unlikely to have any major locomotor abnormality in the lower limbs or lumbar spine.

Inspection of the standing patient

Ask the patient to stand upright with arms outstretched by their sides.

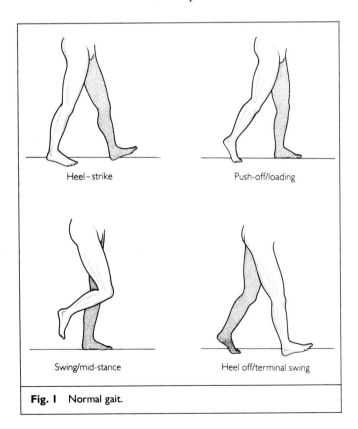

Heel – strike

Push-off/loading

Swing/mid-stance

Heel off/terminal swing

Fig. 1   Normal gait.

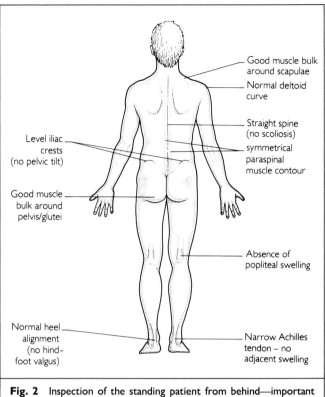

Fig. 2 Inspection of the standing patient from behind—important items to check.

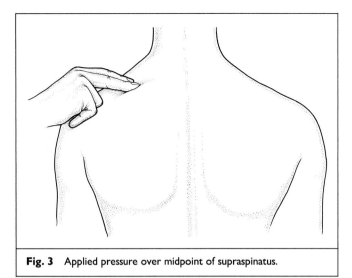

Fig. 3 Applied pressure over midpoint of supraspinatus.

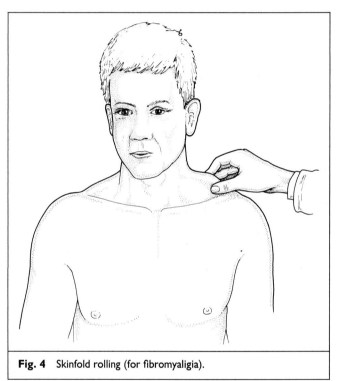

Fig. 4 Skinfold rolling (for fibromyaligia).

1. Inspect from behind (Fig. 2), comparing one side with the other, looking particularly for:

- a straight spine (no scoliosis or rib-cage asymmetry);
- similar level of both iliac crests;
- normal muscle bulk/symmetry, especially around the shoulder and pelvic girdles, and the lumbar spine;
- popliteal swelling;
- swelling/asymmetry around the Achilles tendons;
- hindfoot deformity (valgus/varus).

While in this position apply pressure to the midpoint of each supraspinatus (Fig. 3), and undertake skinfold rolling of overlying skin (Fig. 4) looking for increased tenderness suggestive of fibromyalgia (these being two common sites of involvement).

2. Inspect from the side (Fig. 5), looking particularly for:

- loss of normal cervical and lumbar lordosis, and alteration of normal mild thoracic kyphosis,
- knee deformity (fixed flexion, genu recurvatum, posterior tibial subluxation).

While in this position, test lumbar spine and hip flexion by placing several fingers over the posterior spinous processes of the lower lumbar vertebrae and asking the patient to *bend forwards and touch his or her toes* as best as possible (Fig. 6). The thoracolumbar spine should form a smooth curve and the palpating fingers move apart if the lumbar spine is normal: a good range of movement implies normal hip flexion.

3. Inspect from in front (Fig. 7), comparing one side with the other. Look particularly for:

- swelling, abnormal position, skin change over each sternoclavicular and acromioclavicular joint site;

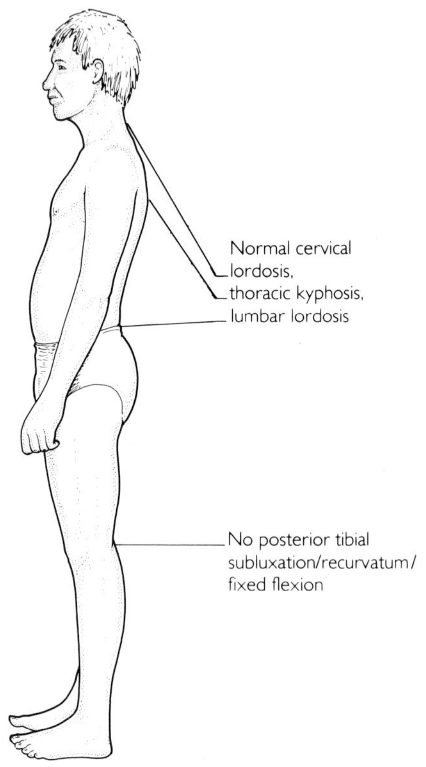

Fig. 5 Inspection of the standing patient from the side—important items to check.

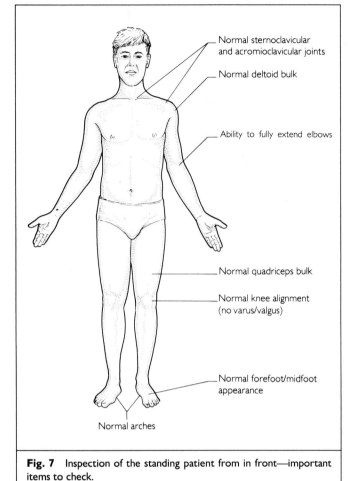

Fig. 7 Inspection of the standing patient from in front—important items to check.

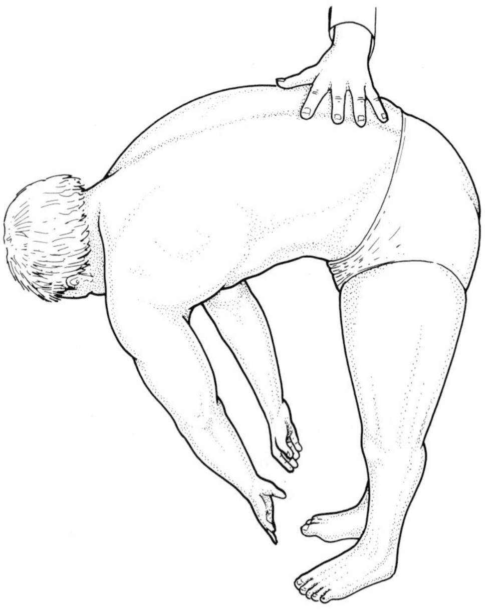

Fig. 6 Inspection/palpation of patients attempting to 'touch the toes'.

- equal shoulder height;
- muscle wasting/asymmetry, especially of deltoids and quadriceps;
- inability to fully extend elbows;
- deformity (particularly varus, valgus) of knee;
- deformity (particularly of hallux, MTPJs) of forefoot and alteration of foot arches (flat feet).

While in this position ask the patient to:

1. *Laterally flex the neck* to each side (Fig. 8), looking for pain or restriction (lateral flexion is a sensitive test for cervical spine abnormality).
2. *Open the jaw wide and move it from side to side* (Fig. 9). It should open easily, without deviation to either side, sufficiently wide to accommodate three fingers vertically.
3. *Place both hands behind the head* with elbows back (Fig. 10). External rotation and abduction are the earliest, most severely affected glenohumeral movements. This action also moves the acromio-clavicular and sternoclavicular joints, and tests the supraspinatus, infraspinatus and teres minor.

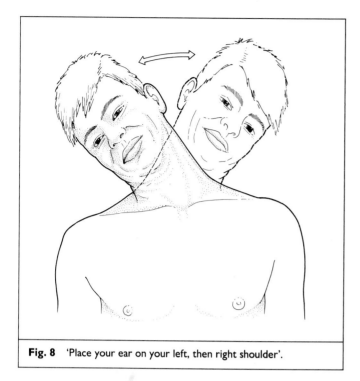

Fig. 8 'Place your ear on your left, then right shoulder'.

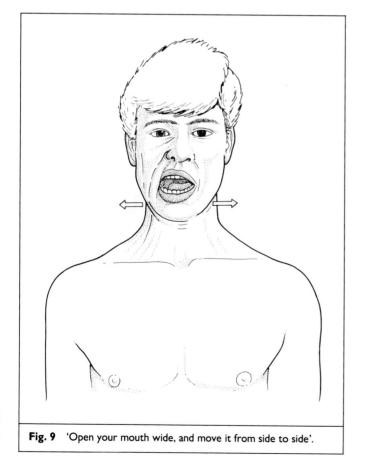

Fig. 9 'Open your mouth wide, and move it from side to side'.

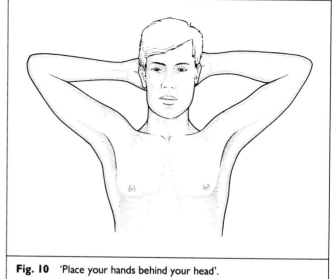

Fig. 10 'Place your hands behind your head'.

4. *Place both hands out in front, palms down, fingers straight*, with elbows at 90° at the side (Fig. 11). Inspect for abnormalities (particularly swelling, deformity, attitude and skin changes) at the distal radioulnar joint, wrists, MCPJs and interphalangeal joints (IPJs). Look for the swelling of extensor tenosynovitis.
5. *Turn the hands over* (supination, Fig. 12, testing proximal and distal radioulnar joints). Inspect the palmar aspects, particularly for wasting, skin changes, flexor tenosynovitis swelling.
6. *Make a tight fist with each hand* (Fig. 13). Observe ability to curl fingers tightly into palms (power grip).
7. *Place the tip of each finger onto the tip of the thumb in turn* (Fig. 14). Observe dexterity for fine precision pinch.
8. *Squeeze across the 2nd to 5th metacarpals* (Fig. 15).

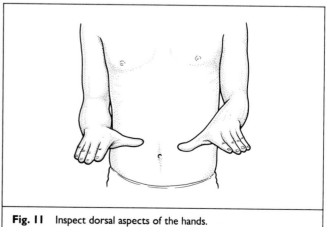

Fig. 11 Inspect dorsal aspects of the hands.

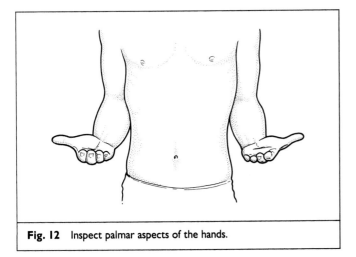

Fig. 12   Inspect palmar aspects of the hands.

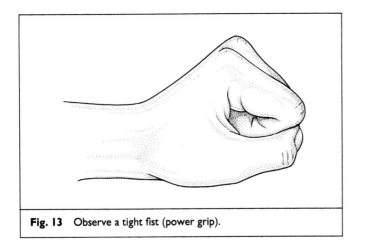

Fig. 13   Observe a tight fist (power grip).

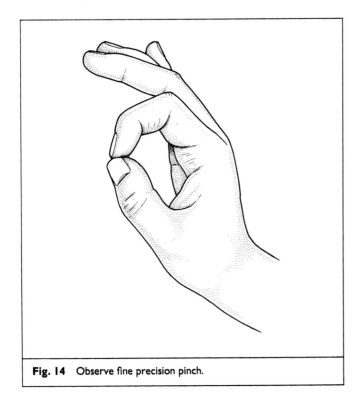

Fig. 14   Observe fine precision pinch.

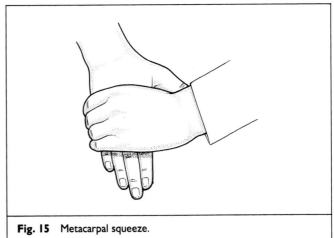

Fig. 15   Metacarpal squeeze.

When asking the patient to undertake such specific actions it is often helpful for the examiner to do the same so that the patient can see exactly what is required (this speeds up the examination considerably).

Inspection/examination of the patient lying on a couch

Elderly patients particularly may find it uncomfortable to lie totally flat, and a sitting up position is adequate for screening manoeuvres. With the patient reclining comfortably:

1. *Flex the hip and knee while holding the knee* (Fig. 16). Ensure normal knee flexion and feel for crepitus. This again tests hip flexion.
2. *Passively internally rotate the hip* with the hip still flexed (Fig. 17). This is a sensitive test for hip disease. Repeat the last two procedures on the other side.

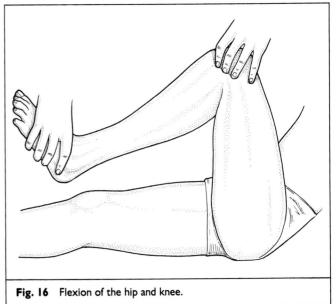

Fig. 16   Flexion of the hip and knee.

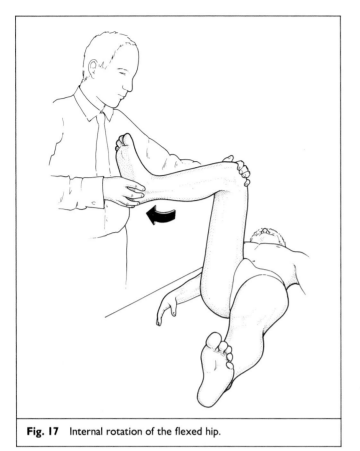

Fig. 17   Internal rotation of the flexed hip.

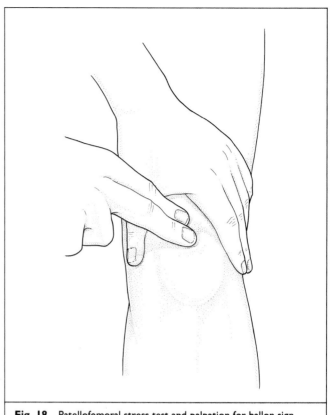

Fig. 18   Patellofemoral stress test and palpation for ballon sign.

3. *Press down on the patella and palpate for a balloon sign in each knee* (Fig. 18). This tests the patellofemoral compartment and for synovitis in a joint commonly affected by all arthropathies.
4. *Squeeze all the metatarsals* (Fig. 19) to test the MTPJs.
5. *Inspect the soles for callosities.*

There are many other simple movements and tests that can be added to such a screen, though if findings for all of the above are normal it is very unlikely, in the face of a normal locomotor history screen, that significant abnormalities will be present. Other features of possible relevance to locomotor disease (e.g. nail changes, clubbing) will have been included in the screening of other systems.

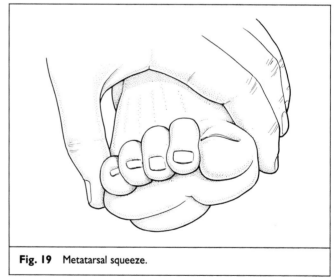

Fig. 19   Metatarsal squeeze.

EXAMINATION OF SPECIFIC REGIONS

1

THE SHOULDER

The principal function of the shoulder is to put the hand into a position where it is able to operate efficiently. Evolutionary development has been accompanied by structural changes in the shoulder girdle and its musculature. The resulting mobility has been acquired at the expense of stability and has led to complexity of soft-tissue components—ligaments, tendons and muscles. Movement is dependent on the unhampered gliding of the periarticular structures—the musculotendinous rotator cuff, the subacromial bursa and the tendon of the long head of the biceps muscles. It is the pathological changes in these structures that cause much shoulder pain.

A great deal can be learned about shoulder function from careful clinical examination and analysis of movement. Normal shoulder motion is the result of a complex of five functional areas: the glenohumeral joint, the acromioclavicular joint, the subacromial joint between the acromioclavicular arch above and the head of the humerus and tuberosities below, the sternoclavicular and scapulothoracic region (Fig. 1).

Shoulder pain is one of the most common medical complaints and a detailed history and physical examination are essential to determine whether shoulder symptoms arise from local injury, or are due to occupation or systemic disease, or result from pain referred from another site. Particular attention should be given to the patient's occupation or sporting activities, and the presence of chronic illness, particularly diabetes mellitus.

Regional shoulder complaints rank fifth among the regional rheumatic diseases as a cause of incapacity or of visiting a physician. Nearly one million cases were recorded in the USA in 1976 by the National Center for Health Statistics (Kelsey, 1982). Data from UK general practices (Department of Health and Social Security, 1986) suggest that approximately 1 in 170 of the adult population will present to their general practitioner

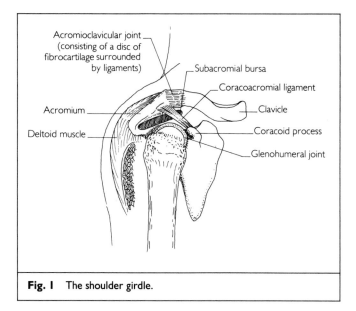

Fig. 1   The shoulder girdle.

with a new episode of shoulder pain each year. This contrasts with 1 in 30 for back pain.

Arthritis of the glenohumeral joint is a relatively infrequent but important cause of shoulder pain. Although the synovial reflections of the joint are extensive, it is very difficult to identify landmarks or localise inflammation to this joint by palpation. Pain or restricted passive external rotation suggests intra-articular diseases and should not be dismissed; it may be associated with systemic disease, for example in inflammatory arthritis or infection.

Disorders of the rotator cuff tendons are common and a large proportion occur in the absence of systemic disease. In these circumstances, local causes, such as chronic repetitive low-grade trauma or excessive and unaccustomed use, either at work or at play, may be responsible. These factors may also cause partial interruption of the blood supply, resulting in incomplete attempts at healing and degeneration, which renders these tissues more vulnerable in the middle-aged and the elderly, in whom the lesions predominate. The pathological hallmarks associated with the rotator cuff syndrome include a spectrum of dystrophic changes in the tendon and accompanying calcification associated with the tendon.

Anatomy

The shoulder joint depends very much on the surrounding soft tissues for its stability and function and the rotator cuff tendons occupy a central role. As they are the site of the majority of lesions producing shoulder pain, knowledge of that anatomy is important in understanding how such lesions may arise and why they affect shoulder function in the way they do.

The shoulder is a multi-axial spheroidal joint between the roughly spherical head of the humerus and the shallow glenoid cavity of the scapula. The shoulder is capable of a great range of movement. It is, however, a potentially very unstable type of joint compared with the hip, which has exact congruity of joint surfaces (Fig. 2). The glenoid labrum of fibrocartilage helps deepen the glenohumeral joint but much of the head of the humerus is still not in continuous contact with the glenoid.

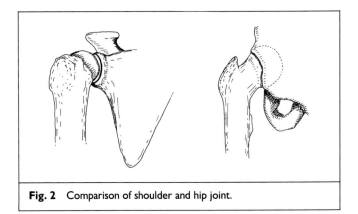

Fig. 2   Comparison of shoulder and hip joint.

Joint capsule, muscles around the shoulder

The capsule of the glenohumeral joint is a synovial-lined, fibrous structure that envelopes the joint. It is loose and allows a 2–3 cm separation of the bones by a distractive force. The intra-articular volume enclosed by the capsule is between 20 and 50 ml. The proximal attachment is to the glenoid and root of the coracoid process, and distally to the anatomical neck of the humerus, with an extension medially 1 cm down the bone shaft. Three minor capsule thickenings, the superior, middle and inferior glenohumeral ligaments help support it. Strength above is provided by the

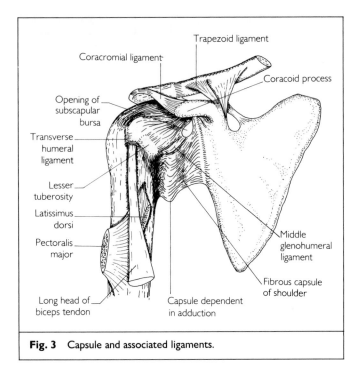

Fig. 3   Capsule and associated ligaments.

rotator cuff tendons. The coracohumeral and transverse humeral ligaments also assist. Below there is no additional support, producing a large inferior recess (Fig. 3). Two or three openings are present in the capsule. Anteriorly is a communication with the bursa behind the tendon of subscapularis and between the tuberosities for the longhead of biceps. Posteriorly an inconstant communication is found with a bursa below the infraspinatus.

Muscles around the shoulder joint

Superiorly lies the supraspinatus, inferiorly there is the long head of triceps, anteriorly is found the subscapularis, whilst posteriorly are the infraspinatus and teres minor. Inside passes the long head of biceps to its insertion on the upper part of the glenoid labrum. The deltoid muscle overlies these tendons. The shoulder joint capsule is fused with parts of the tendons of supraspinatus, infraspinatus, teres minor and subscapularis muscles to produce a musculotendinous cuff, (the rotator cuff) (Fig. 4) although the tendons are fused with the capsule in the adult, they are separate in the newborn. The tendons are very small initially and become lengthened with age. The supraspinatus tendon has a mean length of 19 mm and the infraspinatus and subscapularis a length of 16 mm. The position of the rotator cuff is superiorly over the joint, separating it from the subacromial bursa (no natural communication exists between them).

The supraspinatus muscle is the most important rotator cuff muscle. Arising from the supraspinatus

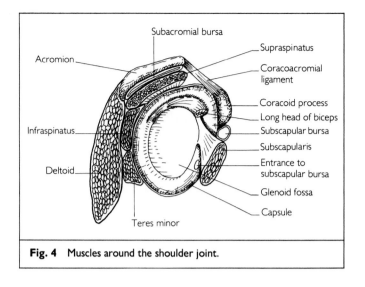

Fig. 4 Muscles around the shoulder joint.

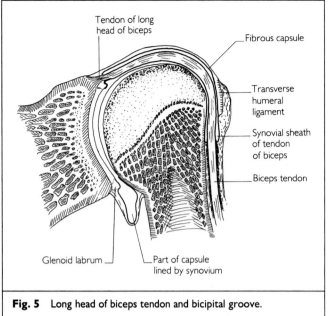

Fig. 5 Long head of biceps tendon and bicipital groove.

fossa of the scapula it inserts into the greater tuberosity of the humerus. As it passes across the superior aspect of the joint, the inferior surface of the tendon merges with the capsule, whilst the superior surface forms part of the floor of the subacromial bursa. The role of this muscle in shoulder movement is controversial: while it assists abduction by fixing the head of the humerus against the glenoid, it is not certain whether or not it is a prime mover. It is generally thought that it is mainly important in the initial 15–20° of abduction, which is otherwise mainly produced by the deltoid muscle.

The infraspinatus muscle has its origin on the posterior aspect of the scapula below the spine and inserts into the greater tuberosity on its posteriosuperior aspect. It is a principal lateral rotator of the humerus.

The teres minor has its origin along the axillary border of the scapula and inserts into the greater tuberosity on its posterioinferior aspect, at which site it is closely associated with the joint capsule and acts to strengthen it. The muscle assists the infraspinatus in its action.

The subscapularis muscle arises from the subscapula fossa and inserts into the lesser tuberosity of the humerus just lateral to the glenoid labrum. The bicipital groove separates it from the rest of the rotator cuff. Within the groove is the long head of the biceps, which inserts into the supraglenoid tubercle (Fig. 5). Often a transverse ligament is present which spans a gap between the tuberosities and forms an additional attachment for the rotator cuff. The subscapularis is important in medial rotation, especially with the humerus in the adducted position.

The rotator cuff tendons and associated capsule insert all round the anatomical neck of the humerus, except inferiorly where only the capsule is attached. In addition to the short muscles, the other principal muscles involved in shoulder movement are the del-

toid, pectoralis major, latissimus dorsi and teres major. Other muscles assist in shoulder movement, for example the triceps and the rhomboid muscles assist with shoulder-girdle movements.

Additional structures around the shoulder

The arch of the acromion covers the superior aspect of the glenohumeral joint and articulates with the clavicle at the acromioclavicular joint. The coracoacromial ligament is a flat band extending from the medial border of the acromion in front of the acromioclavicular joint to the lateral border of the coracoid process of the scapula (Fig. 6).

A number of synovial lined bursae are found around the shoulder joint. There are those associated with the subscapularis and infraspinatus muscles, and in addition bursae are also present over the upper surface of the acromium and between the coracoid process on

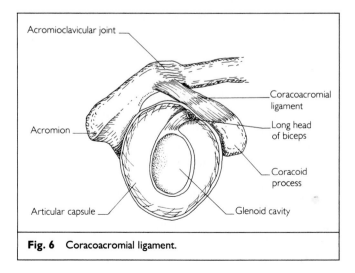

Fig. 6 Coracoacromial ligament.

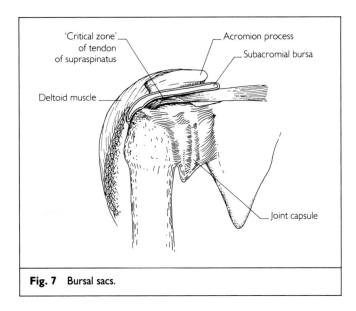

Fig. 7 Bursal sacs.

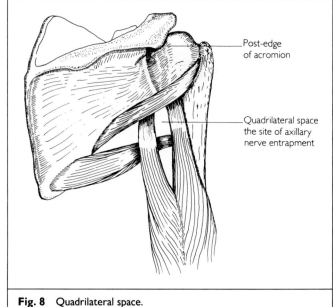

Fig. 8 Quadrilateral space.

the joint capsule. Sometimes bursae are found along the long head of the triceps, the teres major and the latissimus dorsi muscles (Fig. 7). The largest is the subacromial bursa, which laterally is situated between the deltoid muscle and joint capsule, and medially is prolonged under the acromium and coracoacromial ligament, separating these structures from the supraspinatus tendon.

Blood supply to the shoulder
The vessels supplying blood to the shoulder structures are branches of the anterior and posterior circumflex humeral arteries and the suprascapular artery.

Nerve supply to the shoulder
Two main sensory nerves supply the shoulder region. The suprascapular nerve supplies the superior and posterior parts of the joint and capsule and most of the rotator cuff tendon, while the axillary nerve supplies the anterior aspect of the joint and capsule. The axillary nerve arises from the posterior cord of the brachial plexus and exits through the quadrilateral space. This space is bordered superiorly by the teres major, inferiorly by the teres minor, medially by the long head of the triceps, and laterally by the humeral shaft and lateral triceps heads (Fig. 8). After sending a sensory branch to the upper lateral cutaneous surface and a motor branch to the teres minor, the nerve courses anteriorly to innervate the deltoid.

The suprascapular nerve is a branch of the upper trunk of the brachial plexus formed by the 5th and 6th cervical nerves. It passes obliquely beneath the trapezius and crosses the scapula through the suprascapular notch (Fig. 9). The suprascapular nerve has no cutaneous sensory branches but supplies motor branches to the supraspinatus and infraspinatus muscles. The acromioclavicular joint also receives

Fig. 9 Suprascapular notch.

branches from the suprascapular nerve but has a branch from the long thoracic nerve as well.

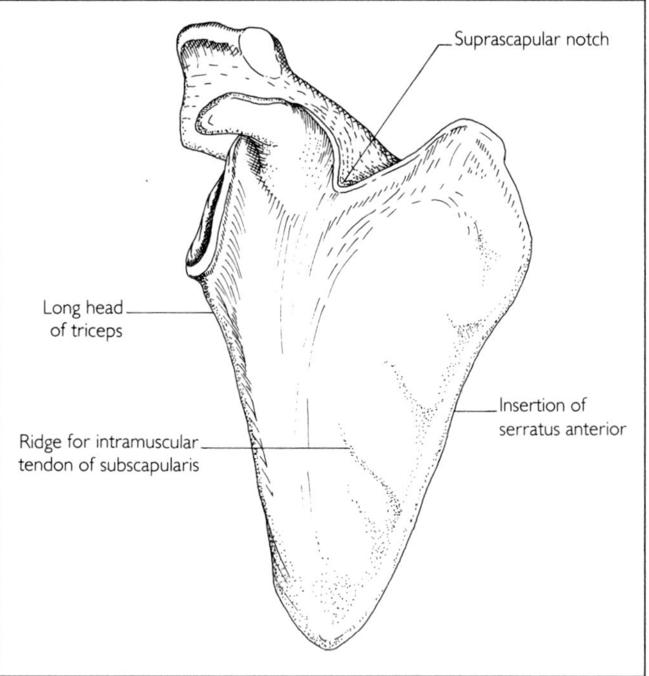

Evolution of the Shoulder

The adoption of an arboreal habitat makes the development of a highly mobile prehensile forelimb useful. The relationship of the scapula to the thorax and the orientation of the humeral head have changed with the evolution of the bipedal primates. As a strut the clavicle is an ancient possession of the vertebrates; it is a dermal bone in origin.

The groups of muscles that perform flexion, extension and adduction of the limb at the girdle show differences in development in the various primates. In quadrupedal primates the emphasis is on flexion, whereas in brachiators it is on adduction. Humans are in some features like brachiators and in others like quadrupedal primates.

Developmental Abnormalities

Congenital elevation of the shoulder (Sprengel's shoulder) occurs when the scapula has only partially descended from the neck of the thorax (Fig. 10). This may be associated with webbing or shortening of the neck.

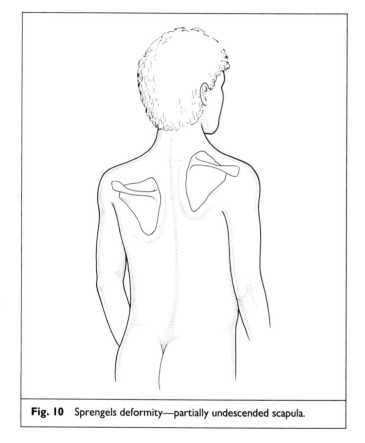

Fig. 10 Sprengels deformity—partially undescended scapula.

Deformity is also seen in Erb's palsy, abduction contracture leading to a sloping deformity or secondary to kyphoscoliosis.

Functional Anatomy of the Shoulder

The structure of the shoulder joint allows an infinite variety of movement but is classically described as having movements of flexion, extension, abduction, adduction, circumduction, and medial (internal) and lateral (external) rotation. The range of movement is greater than in any other joint. In addition, it should be noted that at rest the head of the humerus is retroverted 20–30° from the plane of the trunk; this has implications, for example flexion relative to the trunk must involve some lateral rotation.

Although the glenohumeral joint is the main articulation of the shoulder, it is not the only site of movement. Indeed, despite its greater range, movement of the glenohumeral joint is far less than the overall range of movement, for movement also occurs at four other sites. Scapular rotation may disguise glenohumeral stiffness (Fig. 11), for example. That is not to say that these occur after glenohumeral movement, but they progressively accompany it, allowing the girdle to move in a smooth rhythmic way. The soft-tissue structures of muscles, tendons and ligaments form a complex system which are as important as the bony structures. There are two other joints which also move—the acromioclavicular and sternoclavicular joints. These are true plane joints, but movement does also occur at two other sites which, although not structurally true joints, act like true joints. This movement is between the scapula and thoracic wall and in the subacromial region where the subacromial bursa is found. The bursa acts like a joint space separating the acromioclavicular arch and the head of the humerus. As the subacromial bursa is intimately related to the rotator cuff, the acromioclavicular joint and other nearby skeletal structures, it is often involved when these are the site of a pathological lesion.

The first 30° of abduction is achieved by contraction of the supraspinatus, the next 60° by the deltoid and the final 90° by the trapezius acting on the scapula. Adduction is principally due to the pectoralis major and latissimus dorsi. Forward flexion depends mainly on the pectoralis major and the anterior fibres of deltoid, extension on the latissimus dorsi, teres major and

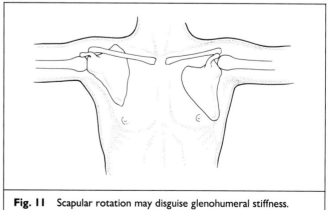

Fig. 11 Scapular rotation may disguise glenohumeral stiffness.

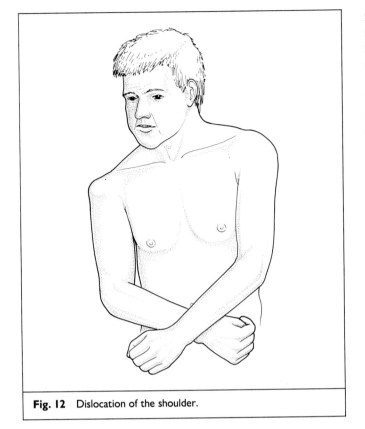

Fig. 12 Dislocation of the shoulder.

the posterior fibres of the deltoid. Lateral rotation is achieved by contraction of the infraspinatus and medial rotation by the pectoralis major latissimus dorsi and the anterior fibres of the deltoid.

Acute stress can result in trauma to the capsulolabral complex of the shoulder and lead to joint subluxation or dislocation (Fig. 12). Symptomatic instability may continue following such episodes; indeed it can develop in the susceptible individual without any history of antecedent trauma. Repeated episodes of instability place increased stress on the stabilising structures such as the rotator cuff and bicipital tendon, thereby giving rise to impingement or tendinitis. In the young athlete, development of tendinitis in the shoulder is such a frequent manifestation of an underlying instability that patients under the age of 25 with shoulder symptoms should always be assessed for the presence of glenohumeral instability.

History

General history

A painful shoulder may be seen in association with several medical conditions and it is therefore important in the evaluation of the shoulder joint to determine whether there is a relevant previous medical history. A previous cerebrovascular accident

may have led to upper limb weakness, spasticity or secondary capsulitis of the shoulder joint, and pain may be referred to the shoulder from those disorders of the upper abdomen which give rise to diaphragmatic and hence phrenic nerve irritation. A Pancoast's tumour at the apex of the lung can present with shoulder-tip pain, and diabetes mellitus has a strong association with adhesive capsulitis. In addition, symptomatic involvement of other joints must be determined at the initial assessment as they may herald the onset of polyarthritis.

There is a close association between disorders of the neck and shoulder, often complicating the diagnosis, and so any history of neck pain or headaches must be recorded, as must a history of intolerance to cold or pallor of the fingers, perhaps indicating Raynaud's phenomenon or thoracic outlet obstruction. A history of previous injury or dislocation of the shoulder and any subsequent treatment to the shoulder is of importance, and in cases where corticosteroid injections have been administered the frequency and location of these need to be established.

Age

The age of the patient may provide clues as to the likely cause of a painful shoulder: for example, osteoarthritis and cervical spondylosis are usually conditions of the elderly. Adhesive capsulitis and degenerative rotator cuff tears tend to occur over the age of 40, and pain resulting from shoulder instability is usually a condition affecting the teenager or young adult. In the case of a rotator cuff tendinitis, the pathology giving rise to the symptoms is to some extent age-related, a rough guide being underlying glenohumeral instability in the under 25-year-old, impingement or tendinitis in the 25- to 40-year-old, and degenerative rotator cuff tendinitis in the over 40-year-old group.

Arm dominance

It is important to establish handedness, as discrepancies in muscle bulk strength and range of shoulder movement may simply reflect the dominance of a particular limb.

Occupational history

Work involving heavy lifting or repetitive movements, especially above shoulder level, may give rise to tendinitis often of insidious onset. Pain is often of an aching nature and muscular in origin, often poorly localised. The patient usually notices the work aggravates or indeed precipitates the symptoms.

Pain history and sources of shoulder pain

Developmentally almost all structures of the shoulder are derived from the C5 sclerotome, at least in part. Therefore pain from any of these deep structures will be perceived in the distribution of the C5 dermatome. This means that pain is localised as much to the insertion of the deltoid and outer aspect of the arm (sometimes extending to the wrist) as the shoulder itself. On the superior aspect of the shoulder is the acromioclavicular joint, which is a structure from the C4 sclerotome, so pain from here is localised to that area and not felt down the arm.

Shoulder pain may either arise from shoulder-related structures or be referred from pathology elsewhere. Local lesions producing shoulder pain may arise from the acromioclavicular joint, the glenohumeral joint itself or the periarticular structures, which the shoulder relies on for its integrity and function. It is important to establish the location of the pain and the presence of night pain or any aggravating or relieving factors. It is also important to establish whether there is associated neck pain as this may indicate the presence of pathology such as cervical spondylosis, which frequently presents with shoulder pain. Whether the onset of pain was acute or gradual should also be established and the relationship of pain to particular activities. Any history of injury or fall is of special relevance.

Location of pain
Pain felt at the tip of the shoulder may be referred from the subphrenic region and pain referred from the cervical spine is often maximal over the superior aspect of the shoulder (Fig. 13). Glenohumeral joint pathology including capsulitis and rotator cuff tears gives rise to deep-seated pain affecting the whole shoulder and often felt to come from the area of the deltoid muscle. It is aggravated by activity and relieved by rest, although it can be a problem at night. Pain from a rotator cuff tendinitis is usually felt at the outer aspect of the upper arm in the region of the deltoid insertion.

Acromioclavicular joint pathology gives rise to a well-localised pain felt at that joint and is aggravated by lying on the shoulder. Sternoclavicular joint symptoms are also well localised. If there is glenohumeral joint subluxation, pain is felt in the anterior or posterior aspect of the glenohumeral joint depending on the direction of the instability, but this is not always so. Pain that radiates up into the neck or into the forearm and hand is suggestive of a cervical or brachial plexus lesion.

Radiation of pain into the arm associated with numbness or paraesthesiae may indicate a compressive neuropathy, and this occurs in thoracic outlet

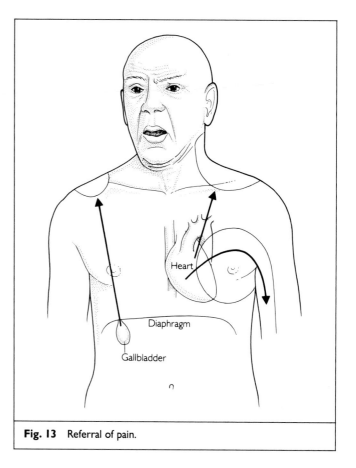

Fig. 13 Referral of pain.

syndrome or suprascapular or axillary nerve entrapments. The pain of a brachial neuritis is usually intense, of acute onset and has a characteristic poorly localised radiation into the arm and shoulder.

Assessing thoracic outlet compression on movement
Thoracic outlet symptoms are aggravated or brought on by activities that involve elevation of the arm. Unlike rotator cuff disorders, however, the symptoms are often aching in nature and tend to radiate into the distal arm, commonly along the ulnar border of the forearm or hand, with associated pallor, coldness or numbness of the fingers.

Axillary nerve entrapment
Entrapment as it passes through the quadrilateral space causes pain, weakness and atrophy. It is usually seen in athletes who carry out excessive overhead activity. Pain is made worse by palpation of the quadrilateral space.

Suprascapular nerve entrapment
The primary symptom is pain, which is described as a deep ache felt over the upper border and body of the scapula. It is well localised and is aggravated by any activity that brings the scapula forward, such as

reaching across the chest. Palpation of the suprascapular notch is tender.

Pain located to the anterior aspect of the shoulder radiating down into the biceps muscle is suggestive of a bicipital tendinitis, especially when found in conjunction with tenderness over the long head of the biceps tendon in the bicipital groove. The tendon becomes prominent when the humerus is externally rotated.

Night pain

Shoulder pain is frequently felt at night. Capsulitis, glenohumeral joint arthritis and chronic rotator cuff tears are associated with a deep-seated constant aching pain which is made worse by changing movement and often wakes the patient. Acromioclavicular joint pathology and rotator cuff tendinitis lead to a more localised pain, which is usually felt when the patient lies on the affected shoulder. With cervical spondylosis pain tends to be less severe at night-time in contrast to pain resulting from shoulder pathology and is often relieved by wearing a soft cervical collar.

Other Symptoms

Stiffness or loss of movement, weakness, numbness, paraesthesiae and headaches also occur with shoulder pain. Stiffness is characteristic of capsulitis and glenohumeral osteoarthritis. The stiffness is often of acute onset in adhesive capsulitis but is more gradual with degenerative arthritis. Weakness when present may be marked. It may be a true weakness or secondary to pain. It occurs rapidly in rotator cuff tears and brachial neuritis or with an entrapment neuropathy, and is mild with associated pain on attempted movement in a rotator cuff tendinitis. When weakness is due to cervical nerve root entrapment it is usually slow and progressive and associated with sensory symptoms. Swelling is not a common complaint but does occur in inflammatory conditions of the acromioclavicular or glenohumeral joints when effusion is present.

Crepitus is often described by the patient as grinding in the shoulder and may indicate subacromial inflammation or acromioclavicular joint or glenohumeral joint arthritis. Clicks, as an isolated symptom, are not infrequent in the normal shoulder. If they are painful then they are significant and are frequently a manifestation of shoulder instability. Clicking sensation produced by certain movements may indicate a glenoid labrum tear or a subluxing biceps tendon.

Instability of the shoulder joint is common and patients may give a history of previous dislocation. Clunks are a feature of major instability. Pain is produced on certain manœuvres, such as throwing, and

there is often a feeling of a dead arm with the latter, which may last for several minutes and be followed by symptoms of rotator cuff tendinitis. Weight training, swimming and throwing sports all have a high incidence of shoulder disorders and, in many cases of glenohumeral subluxation, symptoms are often only noted during sporting activity, particularly in throwing sports.

Examination

A systematic approach is important in order to fully assess all the structures in the joints around the shoulder itself. As with other areas of the musculoskeletal system, it should include an assessment of those areas of the body where a source of referred pain is suspected, such as the upper abdomen in the case of shoulder-tip pain. Both shoulders should be examined, and any difference between the two sides noted, in terms of power, stability and range of motion, taking into the account the handedness of the patient. Neurological examination is important, particularly in cases where cervical spine disease, brachial neuritis or nerve entrapments are suspected; in addition, the peripheral pulses should be examined. Weakness is usually the predominant symptom if there is a primary neurological disorder.

Inspection

Watching the patient remove his or her shirt provides the clinician with the ideal opportunity to observe any functional limitations. Areas of erythema, discoloration, bruising and swelling should be noted. Deformity of the shoulder girdle may be present in acromioclavicular joint separation or fractures of the clavicle or humerus. Muscle wasting, which may be marked if there is cervical root or brachial plexus pathology, is less marked in rotator cuff tears or chronic tendinitis.

Wasting of the supraspinatus or infraspinatus muscles might be noted in chronic tendinitis. Standing behind the patient, the scapulohumeral and scapulothoracic rhythm can be observed as the arms are adducted. The presence of scapula elevation should be noted as this can occur in the presence of a full range of active abduction if there is subacromial or rotator cuff inflammation. Ruptured long head of the biceps tendon can be assessed if the patient is asked to actively contract both biceps muscles with the arms abducted. Pushing against the wall will reveal any winging of the scapula due to weakness of the serratus anterior muscle (Fig. 14) or due to a long thoracic nerve palsy.

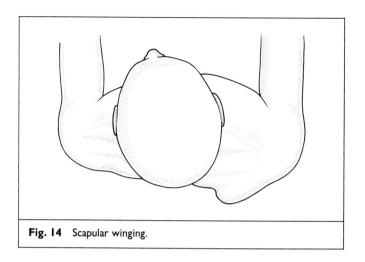

Fig. 14 Scapular winging.

lar joint symptoms commonly occur as a result of instability, and the joint should be examined to assess anterioposterior and inferosuperior laxity. Assessment of glenohumeral joint instability is of particular importance in the young adult presenting with shoulder pain.

When there is swelling around the shoulder it is important to establish whether the fluid lies in the subacromial bursa or in the glenohumeral joint. Communication between the two is occasionally demonstrated by milking the fluid from one compartment to the other. Swelling of the acromioclavicular and sternoclavicular joints are readily palpable and usually tender. The supraclavicular fossa should also be examined for any swelling due to lymphadenopathy or other space occupying lesion.

Palpation

Palpation can establish the presence of any areas of tenderness, assess whether there is joint swelling or determine whether there is any joint instability. The presence of tenderness is an important feature of acromioclavicular and sternoclavicular joint inflammation and it is well-localised over the biceps tendon as it runs in the bicipital groove in cases of bicipital tendinitis. However, in the latter case, the other shoulder should also be examined as the bicipital tendon is normally sensitive to touch. There may be tenderness over the insertion of the infraspinatus, supraspinatus or subscapularis tendon in cases of tendinitis, but in many cases of subacromial pathology no localised tenderness is found. The glenohumeral joint region and the capsular attachment should be palpated, as these areas are tender in instability. The presence of crepitus should be noted and palpation will determine whether or not this is due to inflammation of bursal structures in the subacromial space or due to degenerative changes in the glenohumeral or acromioclavicular joints. Crepitus felt at the scapulothoracic articulation may be due to scapulothoracic bursitis. Examination of the muscles of the shoulder girdle will elicit trigger points of pain, particularly present with myofascial syndromes or isolated muscle spasm.

The sternoclavicular, acromioclavicular and glenohumeral joints should all be assessed for the presence of instability when symptoms appear to be originating from these joints. In the case of the sternoclavicular joint, this can be carried out as the arm moves through full abduction. Pain and tenderness are well localised. In the normal joint the clavicle rotates through 30–40° during this manoeuvre. Excessive widening of the joint as the shoulder is retracted indicates laxity of the sternoclavicular joint capsule and its ligamentous support. Acromioclavicu-

Muscle testing and range of movement (Fig. 15)

Active and passive ranges of movement of both shoulders (Table 1) must be assessed and this should include assessment of abduction, adduction, forward flexion and external rotation, both with the arm by the side and at 90° of abduction (Figs 16–20). Internal rotation is assessed with the elbow extended and the arm at the patient's side. The epicondyles of the humerus are then used as markers for the degree of motion. A combined manoeuvre of internal rotation and extension assesses functional internal rotation and can be demonstrated by asking the patient to put the affected arm behind the back, as in attempting to reach the hip pocket or undo a bra strap (Fig. 21). Measurement is taken by noting the level of the highest spinous process reached by the patient's thumb and comparing this with the unaffected arm.

Limitation of active and passive movement of the shoulder suggests pathology involving the *glenohumeral joint and/or the joint capsule*. Involvement of the glenohumeral joint can occur in isolation or in conjunction with rotator cuff pathology. The latter is seen in many cases of rheumatoid arthritis.

When the glenohumeral joint is involved there is limitation of both active and passive range of movement with pain present on movement, and increasing loss of movement as the joint pathology

Table 1. Range of shoulder movement

Movement	Range
Abduction:	180°
Adduction:	45°
External rotation:	90°
Internal rotation:	90°
Forward flexion:	180°
Extension:	50°

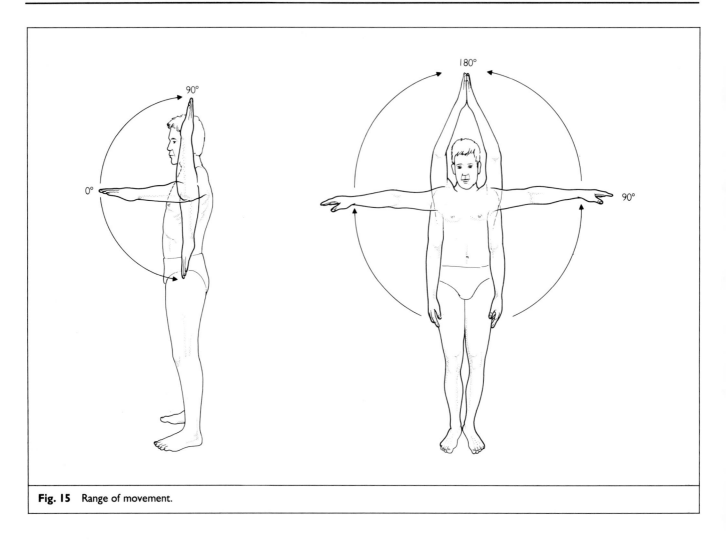

Fig. 15 Range of movement.

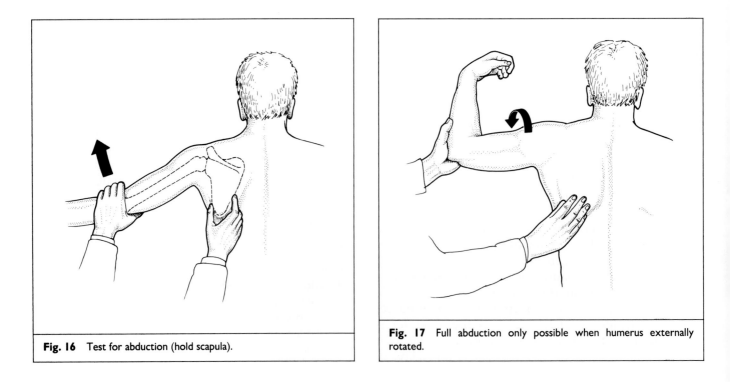

Fig. 16 Test for abduction (hold scapula).

Fig. 17 Full abduction only possible when humerus externally rotated.

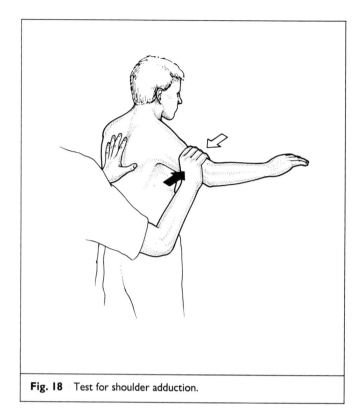

Fig. 18 Test for shoulder adduction.

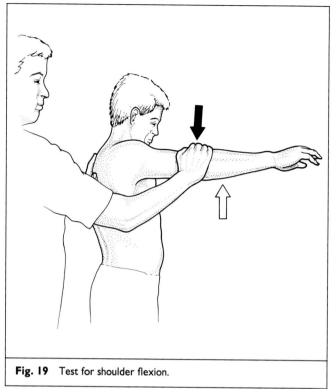

Fig. 19 Test for shoulder flexion.

progresses. Abduction and elevation of the shoulder are the first movements to be lost, and the presence of an effusion should also be noted. There may be warmth and tenderness of the joint when there is inflammation, but large non-inflamed effusions are seen in an apatite-related shoulder arthropathy. Usually other joints are involved as the shoulder is rarely involved alone in inflammatory arthritis, but the shoulder can be involved in isolation when there is a large, complete tear of the rotator cuff. The head of the humerus subluxes in a superior direction and gives rise to an arthropathy involving the subacromial joint.

Active movement may be limited by pain or weakness, and limited active range of movement of the shoulder in the presence of a full passive range of movement of the shoulder implies a disorder of the musculotendinous structures around the shoulder, such as the rotator cuff, and pain tends to be present as a limiting factor in movement. Resisted movements of the shoulder should be tested to assess the involvement of the individual muscles. Resisted abduction should be performed with the arm at the side (Fig. 22) and resisted external rotation and internal rotation (Fig. 23) are also performed in this position with the elbow flexed to 90°. The supraspinatus muscle is best tested with the arm flexed to 30° and abducted to 90° with the arm internally rotated so that the patient's thumb points directly downwards (Fig. 24). Abduction from this position is then resisted by the examiner. Provided any component of adduction is

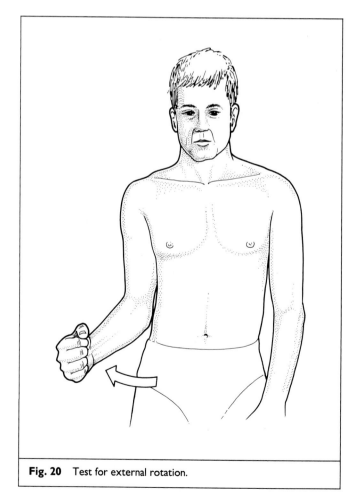

Fig. 20 Test for external rotation.

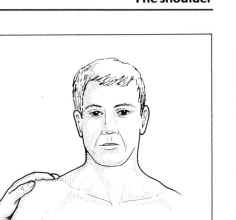

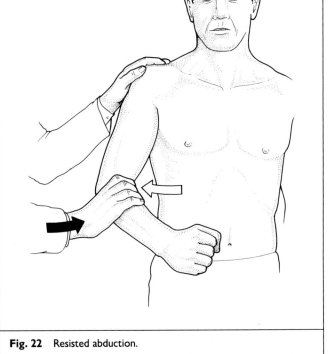

Fig. 21   Test for functional internal rotation.

Fig. 22   Resisted abduction.

the neck, thoracic lesions and intra-abdominal pathology is rarely affected by shoulder movement, whereas pain that is felt only with shoulder movement is usually due to shoulder or thoracic outlet pathology. Pain worsened by neck movement is suggestive of a cervical spine disorder.

When there is inflammation of the glenohumeral joint the pain is felt with most movements of the shoulder, and pain does not disappear in full abduction and elevation as often occurs with subacromial pathology. In the latter condition, the inflamed area is proximal to the area of impingement between the humeral head and under surface of the acromium.

There are several tests that elicit signs of bicipital tendinitis. Yergason's test involves resisted supination of the forearm with the elbow flexed at 90° and held at the patient's side (Fig. 25). In Speed's test the patient flexes the shoulder against resistance with the elbow extended and the forearm supinated (Fig. 26). Both tests are positive if pain is felt in the bicipital groove.

Painful arc of motion

Pain within a definable arc of passive or active motion is usually localised but may be diffuse. It usually indicates a mechanical disorder, such as subacromial impingement, an acromioclavicular arthritis or a

eradicated, resisted internal rotation tests the subscapularis. Resisted external rotation with no element of abduction tests the teres minor and infraspinatus.

Pain on movement

The relationship of pain to movements of the arm and shoulder is helpful in diagnosis, for pain referred from

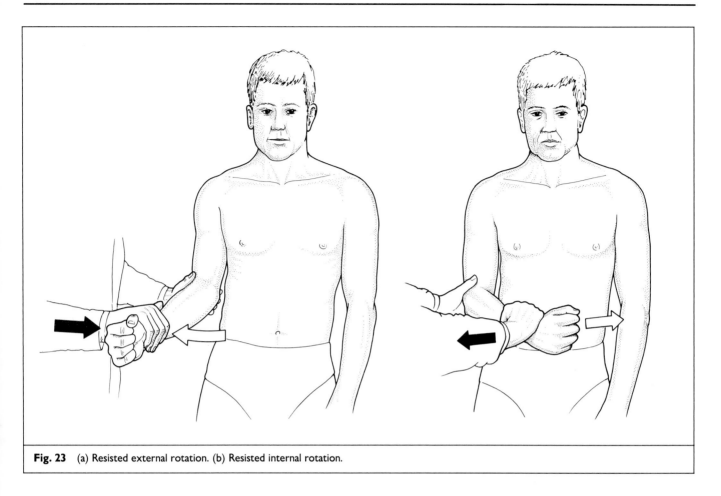

Fig. 23 (a) Resisted external rotation. (b) Resisted internal rotation.

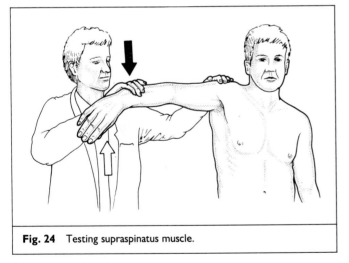

Fig. 24 Testing supraspinatus muscle.

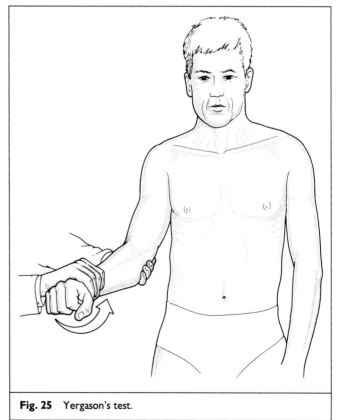

Fig. 25 Yergason's test.

rotator cuff tear. The arc of pain, in terms of both lateral and forward elevation as well as rotation, is frequently an indication of the site of the pathology. If pain occurs during the entire range of glenohumeral motion, it is likely that the source of the problem is in the glenohumeral joint itself. If the arc of pain is from 90° of abduction upwards, it is often the acromioclavicular joint that is the cause of the problem. A painful arc in the middle ranges of motion, with a painless

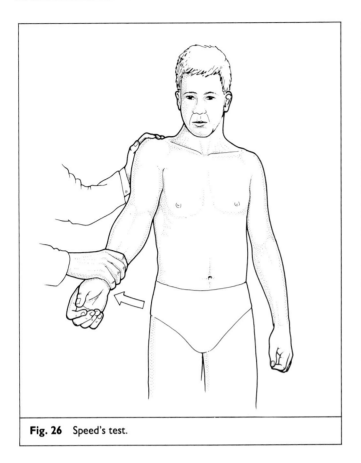

Fig. 26   Speed's test.

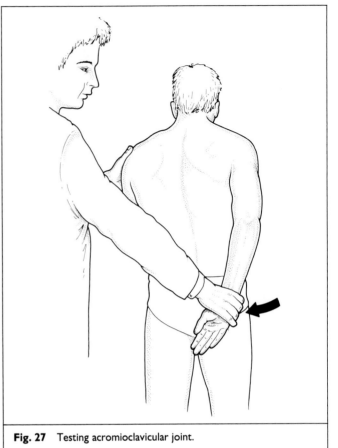

Fig. 27   Testing acromioclavicular joint.

range on either side of the painful arc, is highly sug-gestive of a subacromial pathology, such as a rotator cuff problem or an inferior osteophyte from the acro-mioclavicular joint.

Two manœuvres stress the acromioclavicular joint and produce pain. The patient's arm is held with the elbow extended and then adducted across behind the back and pain is felt over the joint at the limit of adduction in this position (Fig. 27). The other manœu-vre is less specific. It involves bringing the arm across the chest under the chin with the humerus abducted at 90° from the vertical, whilst protracting the shoulder girdle (Fig. 28).

Symptoms of thoracic outlet compression can also be reproduced by several tests. In the costoclavicular test the patient sits with the hands on the thighs and thrusts the shoulder backwards in a bracing movement. Wright's manœuvre involves abduction of the arm from 90 to 180° with the forearm externally rotated. Whilst in this position the neck is rotated to the opposite side and the patient takes a deep breath. During these manœuvres the examiner palpates the radial pulse and a positive test is associated with a decreased or absent radial pulse. These manœuvres, although they may elicit thoracic outlet compression, may give false positive or false negative responses, and it is important to correlate any clinical findings with a reproduction of the patient's symptoms.

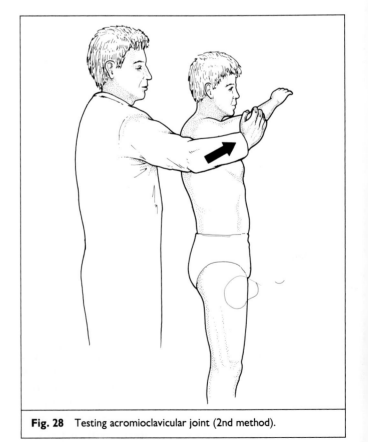

Fig. 28   Testing acromioclavicular joint (2nd method).

Assessing stability

Pain with certain movements, particularly throwing activities in the athlete, may be due to instability. Almost invariably this occurs with the arm in the outstretched (i.e. abducted and externally rotated) or overhead position. Tackling at rugby or throwing a cricket ball are common causes of acute anterior subluxation or instability, presenting as a transiently painful shoulder. The 'dead-arm syndrome' of transient numbness, tingling and weakness of the arm or hand after throwing a ball, with associated pain and later a dull ache is almost pathognomonic of shoulder subluxation. Following acute episodes there is often a history of residual pain and tendinitis lasting several days but usually responding to rest. Instability may be part of a generalised hypermobility and other joints should be examined.

Stability of the glenohumeral joint must be assessed in anterior, posterior and inferior directions. Anterior and posterior stability are best assessed with the patient standing then lying on the examination couch. With the patient standing, the examiner fixes the scapula and shoulder girdle with one hand whilst gripping the humeral head with the fingers of the other. The patient relaxes the arm by the side and the examiner can then attempt to move the humeral head forward and backward in the glenoid fossa. The degree of movement in each direction should be noted and compared with the other shoulder; any palpable clicks may indicate labral pathology.

A more accurate assessment involves the patient lying supine with the shoulder at the edge of the examination couch. The affected arm is supported by the examiner as the other hand fixes the scapula. Movement of the humeral head is then performed by direct pressure. Pain may be produced at the limits of movement. If there is a significant degree of inferior subluxation, a distinct gap can be felt between the humerus and acromium (positive sulcus sign). Laxity of the glenohumeral joint may be present, and further tests are required to determine whether the instability is symptomatic. Testing for anterior instability involves the examiner attempting to extend and externally rotate the affected arm while it is held abducted 90° from the patient's side. The test is positive when there is apprehension on the part of the patient as an external rotation force is applied. With the patient lying supine on the couch and with the arm in external rotation and abduction, force can be applied to the anterior aspect of the upper humerus. This manœuvre often relieves any pain, and the examiner may be able to externally rotate the arm further. If the stabilising force to the anterior aspect of the humerus is removed, the patient feels pain.

Posterior instability can be assessed by stressing the posterior joint capsule, done by applying axial pressure to the forward-flexed, adducted and internally rotated arm.

Pain associated with weakness

Inability to actively abduct the arm occurs in complete tears of the rotator cuff, but usually only in large tears, and wasting of the supraspinatus and especially infraspinatus muscle is often visible and a good indicator of a rotator cuff tear. Several signs have been described to assess the degree of subacromial pathology. One impingement test involves forcing the affected arm up into full forward flexion thereby impinging the rotator cuff against the underside of the anterior acromium (Fig. 29). In another test, the arm is held abducted and flexed at 90° with the examiner supporting the patient's flexed elbow. With the other hand the examiner holds down the patient's shoulder girdle whilst forcibly internally rotating and elevating the affected arm (Fig. 30).

Cervical spine pathology

The cervical spine should always be examined when patients present with shoulder pain. This should involve assessing the range of movement, both active and passive, and assessing muscle strength, areas of muscle spasm and tenderness in the cervical and

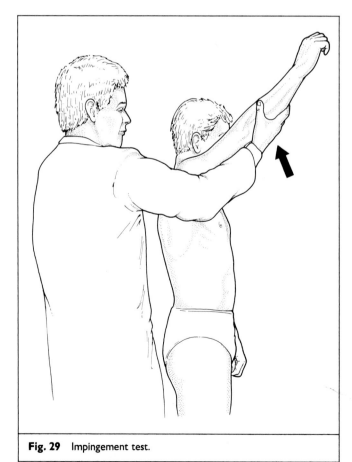

Fig. 29 Impingement test.

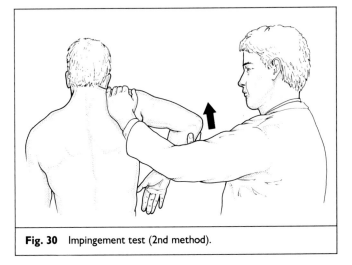

Fig. 30   Impingement test (2nd method).

trapezius regions, and also a neurological examination. Forward flexion, extension, rotation and lateral
flexion need to be assessed and any restriction in
movement noted. Lateral flexion and rotation tend to
be affected early in cervical spondylosis and shoulder
pain resulting from cervical spine pathology may be
reproduced by forced lateral flexion and rotation of the
neck to the affected side.

Further Investigation

Radiographs of the shoulder are frequently normal but
will demonstrate any fractures or degenerative
changes or soft tissue calcium around the shoulder
joint. The integrity of the acromioclavicular joint may
be seen and any underlying subluxation or dislocation
can be reproduced with stress or weight-bearing
views. Arthrography of the shoulder joint is used to
assess the integrity of the rotator cuff. Computerised
tomography is useful in assessing pathology of the
glenoid and glenoid labrum.

Arthroscopy is useful in the diagnosis of instability,
subacromial impingement, rotator cuff tears, shoulder
arthritis, synovitis and intra-articular loose bodies.
Arthroscopy frequently adds important information
to that already obtained by clinical history and examination. Direct visualisation of structures within the
shoulder joint frequently gives information far
superior to that obtained by other diagnostic procedures. This procedure led to a clearer understanding
of the functional anatomy and biomechanics of the
shoulder joint.

Local Aspiration and Injection

Maximum relief of pain is usually achieved with 25–
50 mg of hydrocortisone acetate or equivalent corticosteroid using routine aseptic precautions.

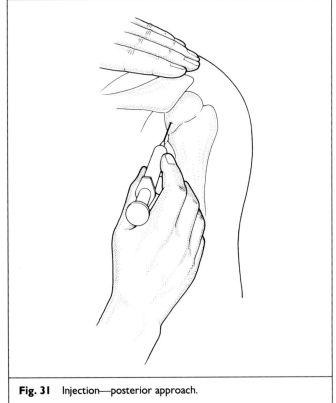

Fig. 31   Injection—posterior approach.

Posterior approach

The most useful technique for non-specialised use is
the posterior approach to the shoulder (Fig. 31). It has
a good chance of success when one is not too sure of
the diagnosis, as it will help in lesions of the supraspinatus, infraspinatus and subscapularis tendons, and
in disorders of the glenohumeral joint.

The patient sits with his or her back to the doctor
who palpates the spine of the scapula, following it
laterally until it turns forward to become the acromium
process, and then with the forefinger finds the coracoid process. The line between the two marks the track
of the needle. If the needle is advanced 1 inch below
the acromium process there is no resistance and the
top of the needle is in the upper recess of the shoulder
joint, away from the head of the humerus and the
cartilage of the glenoid cavity.

Lateral approach

This is the best approach for treating a supraspinatus
tendinitis (Fig. 32). The patient is seated with the arm
loosely at his or her side; the arm is not rotated.

Palpate the most lateral point of the shoulder and
advance the needle medially below the acromium process and slightly posteriorly along the line of the
supraspinous fossa. Inject when 1 inch of the needle is

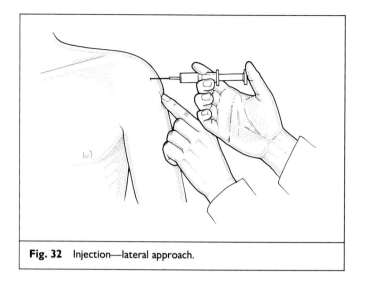

Fig. 32 Injection—lateral approach.

inserted. It is important that the patient does not tense the muscle, as it may then be difficult to inject.

Anterior approach to the shoulder

This approach is a little more difficult (Fig. 33). If the patient lies on his or her back with the forearm laid across the abdomen, the shoulder is partially internally rotated. It is now possible to feel the coracoid process and the injection should be given just lateral to this in the direction of the joint-line. Passive rotation of the arm will easily identify the head of the humerus.

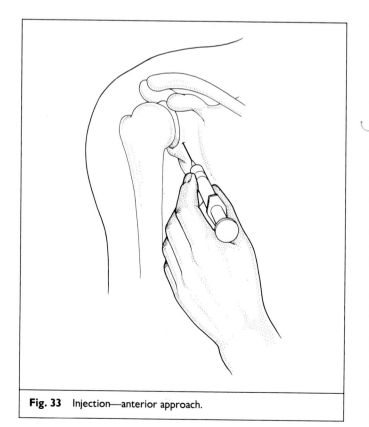

Fig. 33 Injection—anterior approach.

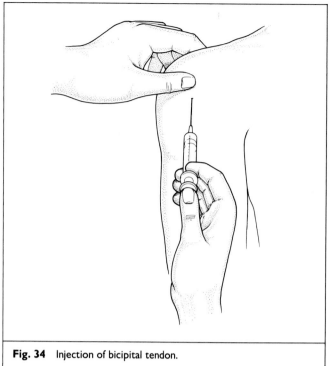

Fig. 34 Injection of bicipital tendon.

The acromioclavicular joint

The joint is a plane articulation and therefore it is possible to inject it certainly from in front (Fig. 34). Pain arising from the joint is associated with tenderness on palpation and occasionally with swelling. The joint cavity is small and will seldom accept more than 0.5 ml of fluid. Acute lesions often settle with rest alone.

Sternoclavicular and sternomanubrial joint

With careful palpation these can be located and injected.

The glenohumeral joint

This is the true shoulder joint, and the main physical sign of glenohumeral disease is limitation of external rotation of the arm. The glenohumeral joint is best approached from the posterior or anterior aspect. The ease of injection should determine whether the needle is in the right place.

Injections of steroid into this joint can help the pain of the frozen shoulder and also reduce inflammation in inflammatory joint conditions.

Bicipital tendinitis

Treatment is the same as for other muscular tendinous lesions. Injection of the tendon sheath with hydrocortisone should be performed with care, as injection of the tendon may lead to rupture.

The tendon is tender and is easily palpated in the bicipital groove of the humerus. The site of maximum tenderness is marked and a needle inserted into the sheath at this mark and 0.5 ml injected. The needle is then directed superiorly along the tendon, in the sheath, for about 2 cm and more material injected. The needle is then partially withdrawn and redirected inferiorly and the remainder of the steroid injected.

Pain spots around the shoulder

Anatomical areas which are rich in pain nerve endings include the muscle–bone and ligament–bone junctions. Most pain spots around the shoulder are at these entheses. The tender areas are usually located along the scapula margin or along the spine of the scapula. They frequently respond to a weak lignocaine–corticosteroid mixture (e.g. hydrocortisone 10 mg diluted with 5 ml of 1% lignocaine). Painful tender spots around the shoulder are often referred from the neck, and in these patients the discomfort is unrelated to shoulder movements.

2

THE ELBOW

As part of the upper limb complex, the primary role of the elbow is to permit and assist accurate spatial positioning of the hand. The elbow anchors the strong flexors and extensors of the wrist and hand, and once the shoulder has directed the hand in a gross, stable fashion, co-ordinated elbow movements permit fine adjustments to limb height and length. In addition, forearm rotation, at both elbow and wrist, helps place the hand in the most effective functional position.

Frequent demands on forearm muscles and poor soft-tissue protection make elbows particularly prone to enthesopathy and bursitis. The elbow is an uncommon primary target site for arthritis other than haemophilia- and syringomyelia-associated Charcot's arthropathy. Although quite commonly involved in inflammatory arthropathies (e.g. rheumatoid, psoriasis) primary osteoarthritis of the elbow, other than in the subset of pyrophosphate arthropathy, is distinctly unusual.

Functional Anatomy

The elbow is a compound joint comprising three articulations: the humeroulnar and humeroradial joints (permitting flexion/extension), and the proximal radioulnar joint (which with the humeroradial and inferior radioulnar joint permits rotation; Fig. 1).

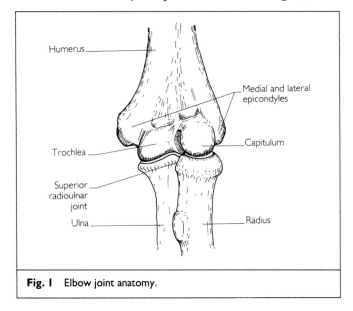

Fig. 1 Elbow joint anatomy.

The **humeroulnar ('trochlea') joint** forms a uniaxial hinge between the trochlea of the humerus and the ulna trochlea notch. When the elbow is fully flexed (*c.* 145°), the longitudinal axes of the upper arm and forearm are parallel. However, due to the inclined contour of the trochlea, as the arm extends in the anatomic position (palms facing anteriorly) the long axes of the upper arm and forearm form a valgus 'carrying angle' at the elbow (Fig. 2). This is wider in females (10–15°) than in males (5°) and may be increased—cubitus valgus—as a developmental abnormality (e.g. as part of Turner's syndrome). The opposite—cubitus varus—is a less common developmental anomaly.

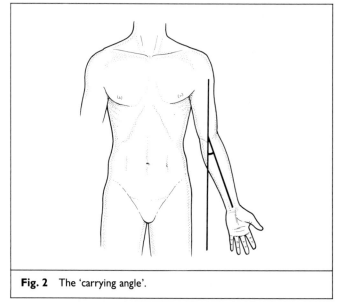

Fig. 2 The 'carrying angle'.

The **humeroradial joint** is a modified uniaxial hinge (allowing rotation as well as flexion/extension) corresponding in form to a ball and socket between the capitulum of the humerus and the concave fovea of the radial head. During supination/pronation the radial head revolves on the capitulum.

The **superior radioulnar joint** comprises the pivot joint between the proximal rim of the radial head and the ulnar radial notch, together with the cartilage-lined annular ligament which encircles the radial

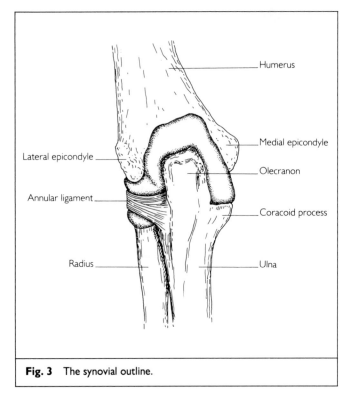

Fig. 3   The synovial outline.

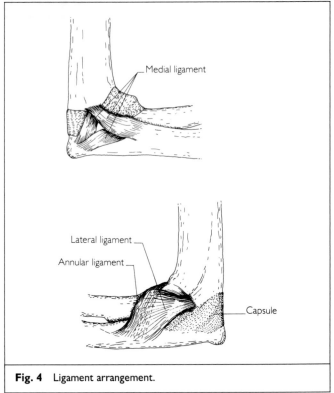

Fig. 4   Ligament arrangement.

head. The very strong interosseous membrane of the forearm prevents parallel displacement of the ulna and radius, and transmits longitudinal stresses from one bone to the other.

The three elbow joints share a common capsule, thus presenting an extensive synovial volume (Fig. 3). Both humeral epicondyles are extracapsular, but the olecranon, coronoid and radial fossae of the humerus, and the tips of the olecranon and coronoid process, are within its confines. Beneath the annular ligament the capsule extends as the sacciform recess. There are large intracapsular fat pads in each of the three fossae of the humerus which, together with muscle and soft tissues, help buttress against extremes of movement. Stability is afforded by the tight-fitting trochlear joint, the annular ligament, the cord-like radial collateral ligament and the fan-shaped ulnar collateral ligament (Fig. 4). The last of these has two parts which, along with flexor carpi ulnaris, form the cubital tunnel through which passes the ulnar nerve. The capsular pattern of restriction is greater limitation of flexion than extension, with equal limitation of supination and extension.

The axis of flexion/extension runs through the humeral epicondyles: all muscles passing in front of this axis act as flexors, all those passing behind as extensors. Many of these muscles act on several joints and their action at the elbow is dependent on the attitude of neighbouring joints. The principal flexors of the elbow (Fig. 5) include:

- *Biceps:* joining the scapula to the radial tuberosity, thus supinating as well as flexing the elbow.
- *Brachialis:* a short muscle between the distal humerus and ulnar tuberosity, acting as a strong pure flexor.
- *Brachioradialis:* joining the lateral humerus to the radial styloid process, bringing the forearm into the neutral rotation position and then flexing the elbow.

The principal elbow extensor is the triceps, joining the scapula (via its long-head origin) and humerus (via medial and lateral heads) to the olecranon, acting to extend the elbow and swing the arm backwards (Fig. 6). Pronation is principally via the proximal pronator teres (the anterior interosseous nerve passes between the two heads of this muscle) and the distal pronator quadratus. Although the biceps is the strongest supinator in flexion, the supinator muscle acts in any flexion/extension position (in 30% of people the posterior interosseous nerve passes through the fibrous arcade of Frohse between the two heads of supinator and may rarely become compressed—*radial tunnel syndrome*—causing weakness of forearm extensors but no sensory loss). The elbow can normally undergo approximately 145° of active flexion from the fully extended position; passive flexion can often achieve another 10–15°. The elbow hyperextends 10° in many normal women (greater extension may reflect hyper-

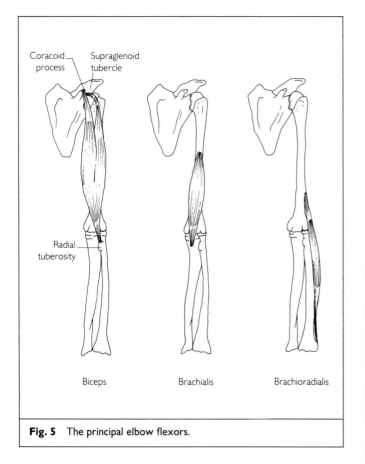

Fig. 5 The principal elbow flexors.

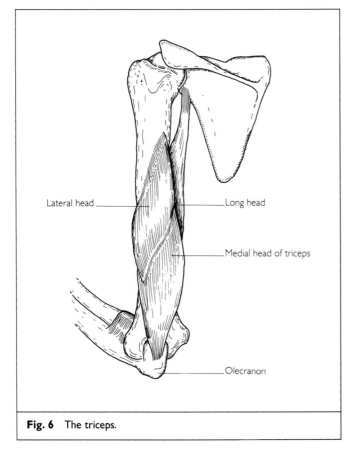

Fig. 6 The triceps.

mobility syndrome). Individuals with well-developed muscles may lack 10° at both ends of the range.

The bones and ligaments around the elbow act to anchor the origins of the forearm muscles. The origins of the extensores carpi radialis brevis and longus (the 'fist clenchers') at the lateral epicondyle (with brachioradialis originating just above) are the usual site of pain in *lateral epicondylitis* (Fig. 7). Both muscles are weak elbow flexors but more importantly they extend the wrist, optimising the action of the flexors and thus permitting maximal power grip. The common tendon insertion at the medial epicondyle (for pronator teres, flexor carpi radialis, palmaris longus, flexor carpi ulnaris) is similarly the site of pain in 'medial epicondylitis' (Fig. 8).

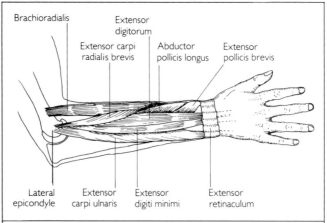

Fig. 7 Extensor insertion at the lateral epicondyle.

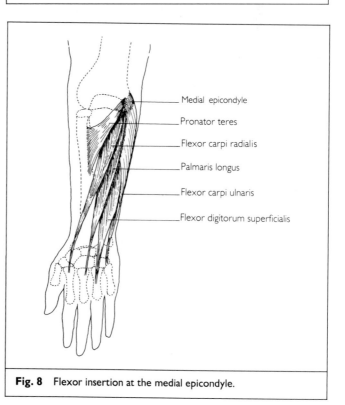

Fig. 8 Flexor insertion at the medial epicondyle.

Several bursae, none of which communicate with the joint, may occur around the elbow, the largest and clinically most important being the superficially placed olecranon bursa overlying the olecranon prominence.

Symptoms

Pain from the three elbow compartments is usually felt maximally at the elbow close to the site of origin: severe arthropathy may cause radiation of pain down the forearm and to a lesser extent back up to the upper arm. The pain of lateral epicondylitis ('tennis elbow') is usually maximal close to the epicondyle, radiating down the outer aspect of the forearm towards the wrist (Fig. 9); it is particularly marked during power grip with the wrist extended. Medial epicondylitis ('golfer's elbow') causes maximum pain around the medial epicondyle radiating down the flexor aspect of the forearm towards the wrist (Fig. 9). Pain from olecranon bursitis is well-localised and usually shows no clear relationship to passive or resisted elbow movement: it may be provoked by leaning the elbow on a table, or on flexion at the elbow only when tight clothing is worn (e.g. a coat).

Four dermatones cover sensation around the elbow (Fig. 10): C5/6 on the radial side and T1/2 on the ulnar side. Pain referred from above is usually ill-defined at the elbow with the site of maximum intensity elsewhere; it can be from glenohumeral or rotator cuff lesions, and from root entrapment (C5 or C6; less commonly T1, T2). Pain may be referred up towards the elbow from De Quervain's tenosynovitis, carpal tunnel syndrome or occasionally severe wrist arth-

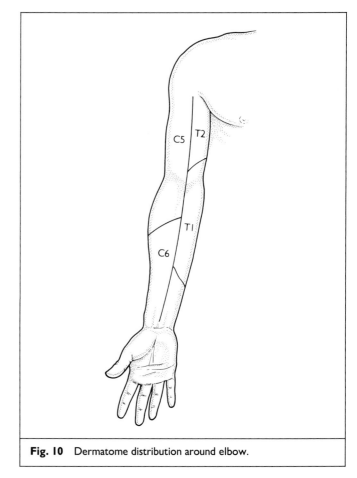

Fig. 10 Dermatome distribution around elbow.

ropathy (particularly with a proximal synovial extension or Baker's cyst).

Examination

Inspection

Inspection from in front and behind the elbow with the patient's arm hanging by his or her side is followed by inspection during active flexion, extension and supination/pronation.

In the posterior view (Fig. 11) the most prominent feature is the olecranon process: para-olecranon grooves separate this from the epicondyles, the medial epicondyle being more prominent than the lateral (the three bony prominences form a straight line with the elbow extended). Anteriorly the triangular cubital fossa (Fig. 12) forms a hollow bounded superiorly by the biceps and its tendon, medially by the pronator teres and the common flexors, laterally by the brachioradialis, and the floor comprising the brachialis muscle and tendon (plus joint capsule and supinator). The fossa contains the brachial artery and veins, the median and musculocutaneous nerves, and superficially the median cubital vein (joining the medially placed basilic to the cephalic vein).

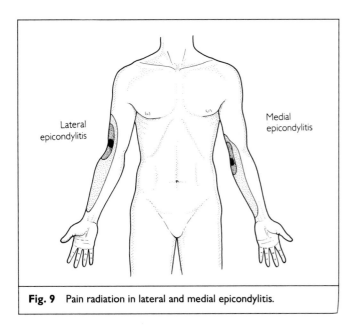

Fig. 9 Pain radiation in lateral and medial epicondylitis.

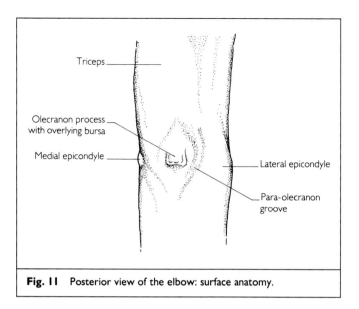

Fig. 11 Posterior view of the elbow: surface anatomy.

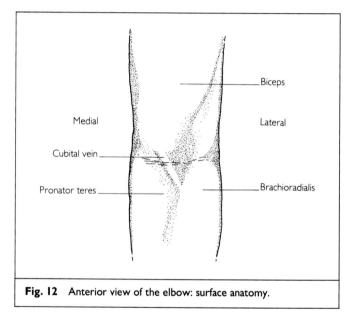

Fig. 12 Anterior view of the elbow: surface anatomy.

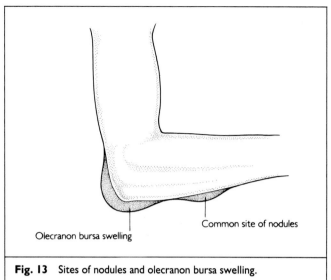

Fig. 13 Sites of nodules and olecranon bursa swelling.

Inspect the skin for erythema (confined to bursitis or over the whole joint), scars and other changes, including psoriasis (the extensor aspect is a common site). The extensor forearm surface and olecranon are also common target sites for nodules and pressure sores (Fig. 13).

Synovial swelling may be apparent over the radial head anteriorly, and posteriorly over the para-olecranon groves (medial > lateral). With marked synovitis the whole elbow region may appear swollen. Olecranon bursitis produces localised smooth swelling around the olecranon prominence (Fig. 13); nodules within it may produce a lumpy contour.

As the patient actively flexes and extends the elbow, the main deformities to look for are fixed flexion (inability to fully extend the elbow), cubitus valgus or varus (assessed with the elbow extended), and poster-ior subluxation of the olecranon on the humerus. The resting attitude may suggest the degree of discomfort or presence of joint disease. A capsular pattern of restriction usually affects flexion more than extension, with supination/pronation affected last: in the presence of synovitis/effusion the patient is therefore most comfortable with the elbow positioned in flexion (c. 45–70°).

Ask the patient to supinate and pronate the hands with the elbows tucked into his or her side at 90° flexion (Fig. 14). If the proximal or distal radioulnar

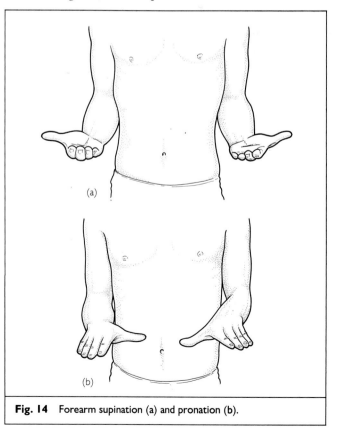

Fig. 14 Forearm supination (a) and pronation (b).

joints, or the humeroradial joint, are compromised these movements may be painful and/or reduced (usually equally): the patient often undertakes a trick manœuvre, adducting the elbow across the abdomen to rotate the ulnar and thus increase supination.

Palpation

The elbow is conveniently palpated with the examiner standing behind the patient with the patient's shoulder extended so that the elbow points backwards in mild flexion (Fig. 15). Pass the back of the hand over the extensor surface of the distal upper arm, elbow and forearm to feel for increased temperature over the para-olcranon grooves and olecranon bursa. The landmarks of the medial and lateral epicondyles are easily felt. On the medial side, feel for the ulnar nerve below the epicondyle for thickening and disproportionate tenderness (this is the commonest site for ulnar nerve entrapment). The medial supracondylar lymph nodes may be palpable if enlarged. Palpate for nodules (even if not immediately apparent) along the extensor forearm border. Palpate for swelling of the olecranon bursa with the arm in extension: if the arm goes into flexion the bursa will become more tense and prominent. A balloon sign will confirm a moderate to large fluid collection. Synovitis will produce soft-tissue swelling in the two para-olecranon grooves, particularly on the medial side: firm palpation at these sites may produce capsular tenderness.

Place a thumb and two fingers of one hand over the olecranon, medial epicondyle and lateral epicondyle. In extension the three fingers will form a straight line, whereas in flexion the fingers will form the points of an equilateral triangle (Fig. 16). Loss of such symmetry on flexion implies loss of height at the elbow due to cartilage and bone attrition ('triangle' sign). Place a finger in each para-olecranon groove to feel for crepitus from the humeroulnar and humeroradial joint while the patient flexes or extends.

Coming to the front of the patient, palpate over the radial head region for soft-tissue swelling due to synovitis. Occasionally palpable anterior synovial extensions may almost fill the cubital fossa (predisposing to partial radial nerve palsy due to pressure on the posterior interosseous nerve). Pressure over the radial head may produce capsular/joint line tenderness, and if there is associated joint damage and annular ligament laxity there may be excessive movement of the radial head with crepitus. Keeping the thumb over the radial head region, passively supinate and pronate with the other hand (thumb placed over ulnar styloid region) to detect crepitus (both joints) and assess the range of passive movement, and enquire concerning pain (Fig. 17). Pass the back of the hand down the flexor aspect of the distal upper arm, elbow and forearm, again feeling for increased temperature, particu-

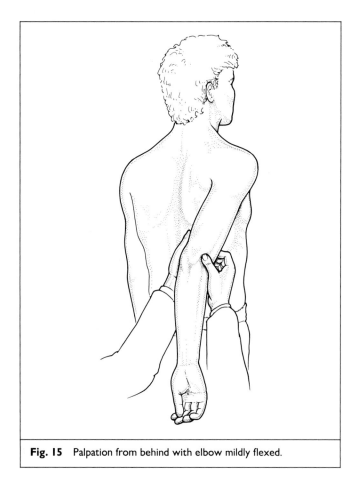

Fig. 15 Palpation from behind with elbow mildly flexed.

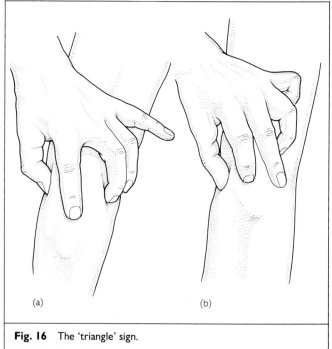

(a)   (b)

Fig. 16 The 'triangle' sign.

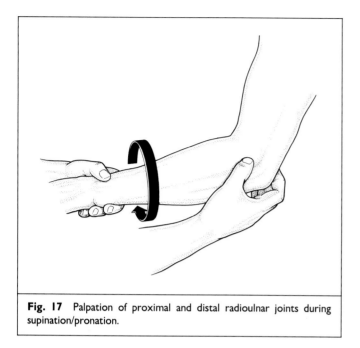

Fig. 17 Palpation of proximal and distal radioulnar joints during supination/pronation.

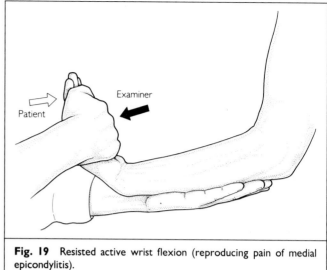

Fig. 19 Resisted active wrist flexion (reproducing pain of medial epicondylitis).

larly over the radial head region. The range of passive flexion and extension is assessed (looking particularly for restriction ± stress pain) and compared with active movements; similar restriction suggests synovitis, a greater passive range favours a neuromuscular rather than joint cause.

Additional tests

Tennis elbow (lateral epicondylitis): palpate over the common extensor origin at the lateral epicondyle. This may produce marked tenderness: in some cases tenderness is more distal occurring over the radial head region. Confirmation is by resisted active wrist extension which reproduces the pain of which the patient complains (Fig. 18).

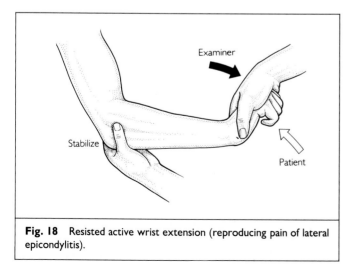

Fig. 18 Resisted active wrist extension (reproducing pain of lateral epicondylitis).

Golfer's elbow (medial epicondylitis) frequently gives tenderness over the medial epicondyle at the insertion site of the wrist flexor/pronator group (pronator teres, flexor carpi radialis, palmaris longus, flexor carpi ulnaris). Resisted active wrist flexion with the hand supinated will reproduce the pain (Fig. 19).

Collateral ligament stability may be tested as follows. Flex the patient's elbow to *c.* 20–30° and, holding the elbow in one hand, apply a progressive varus force (to test the lateral ligament) and then a valgus force (to test the medial ligament) on the distal forearm (Fig. 20), noting any pain or increased lateral movement.

Muscle power, if required, can be assessed by resisted active movements with the patient's arm adducted to the side and the elbow positioned at 90°. Firmly holding the elbow with one hand and the distal forearm with the other (power grip) ask the patient to:

1. *push out in extension*—principally triceps (radial nerve, C7), and then
2. *pull upwards to the shoulder in flexion*—principally biceps and brachialis (both musculocutaneous nerve; C5/6); still holding the elbow, grasp the distal forearm along its longitudinal axis and ask the patient to:
3. *supinate against resistance*—principally biceps (musculocutaneous nerve; C5/6) and supinator (radial nerve; C6); and then
4. *pronate against resistance*—principally pronator teres (median nerve; C6), and pronator quadratus (anterior interroseous branch; C8/T1).

Nerve entrapment may affect the ulnar (most common by far, median or radial nerves. Helpful tests include:

- *Tinel's sign:* light percussion over the ulnar nerve

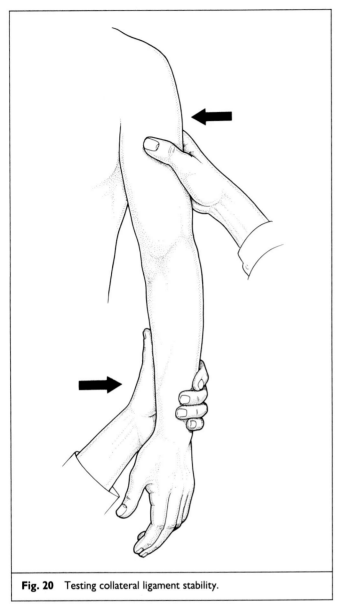

Fig. 20   Testing collateral ligament stability.

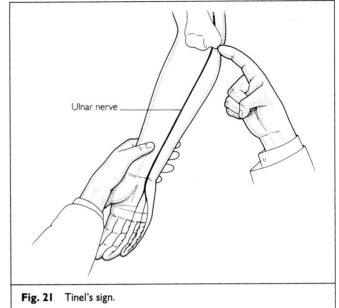

Fig. 21   Tinel's sign.

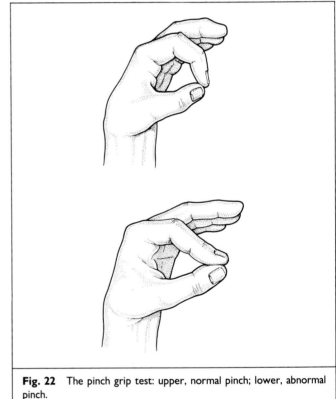

Fig. 22   The pinch grip test: upper, normal pinch; lower, abnormal pinch.

as it travels through the medial para-olecranon groove produces tingling in an ulnar distribution in the forearm/hand distal to the point of compression (Fig. 21). The most distal point at which the abnormal sensation is felt can be used to indicate the limit of nerve regeneration (serial testing can therefore crudely reflect rate of regeneration).

● *Elbow flexion test:* the patient holds the elbow in full flexion for 5 minutes. Tingling in an ulnar distribution again suggests a cubital tunnel syndrome.

● *Pinch grip test:* the patient attempts to oppose the tips of the index finger and thumb. If the normal tip-to-tip pinch is replaced by a pulp-to-pulp pinch (Fig. 22), reflecting impairment of index finger and thumb flexors, entrapment of the anterior interosseus nerve (a branch of the median nerve) as it passes between the two heads of pronator teres is

suggested (*anterior interosseous nerve syndrome*). If the median nerve is compressed just prior to the anterior interosseous division, the flexor carpi radialis, palmaris longus and flexor digitorum muscles are also weak (*pronator teres syndrome*). In both cases, there is sensory impairment in a median nerve distribution. Rarely (1% of people) the median nerve is compressed as it passes (± the brachial artery) beneath the ligament of Struthers, an anomalous band running from a spur on the humerus to the medial epicondyle: in this case (*humerus supracondylar process syndrome*) the pronator teres is also involved (± vascular, as well as neurological, symptoms).

Local Aspiration and Injection

Elbow joint

The two easiest approaches to the joint are anterolaterally and posteriorly. With either approach, fluid aspiration and ease of injection both confirm correct positioning.

Anterolateral approach, towards the humeroradial joint line

Fluid usually accumulates earliest and most prominently anteriorly around the radial head (large synovial extensions, particularly in rheumatoid arthritis, may indeed expand anteriorly to fill much of the cubital fossa). With the patient's elbow resting on a firm comfortable surface, and held flexed at 90°, palpate the head of the radius while passively supinating and pronating the patient's forearm. The joint-line should be readily identified, and associated soft-tissue/fluid swelling is commonly palpable at this site. Pass the needle tangentially in towards the joint line from a superolateral angle (Fig. 23), aiming to place the tip just within the capsule rather than deep between the two bones.

Posterior approach, towards the olecranon fossa

Fluid also expands posteriorly to cause swelling that may be apparent in the para-olecranon grooves (medial > lateral). Again with the patient's elbow

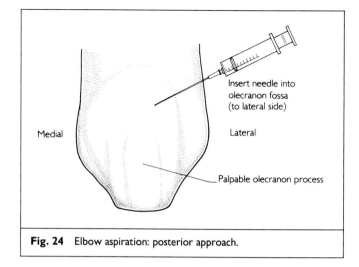

Fig. 24   Elbow aspiration: posterior approach.

flexed to 90° and comfortably supported, identify the olecranon process (receiving the indistinctly felt triceps tendon), the para-olecranon grooves and the olecranon fossa. Insert the needle above the superior aspect of the olecranon, slightly to the lateral side, just into the olecranon fossa (Fig. 24).

Lateral epicondylitis ('tennis elbow')

Injection is into the site of maximal tenderness. In the majority of cases this is the anterior part of the epicondyle at the extensor carpi radialis brevis origin; less commonly it is the supracondylar crest (exensor carpi radialis longus origin), or more distally where extensor carpi radialis brevis overlies the radial head (Fig. 25). The patient is positioned with the forearm supported and the elbow in mid flexion. Having identified the maximally tender site, the needle is aimed vertically downwards until it touches bone. Slightly withdraw the needle, then infiltrate both deeply (as near as possible to bone) and more superficially using a fan

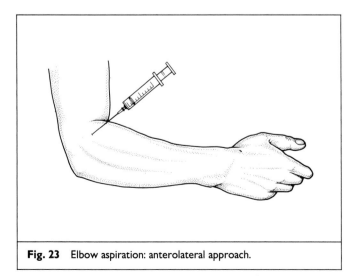

Fig. 23   Elbow aspiration: anterolateral approach.

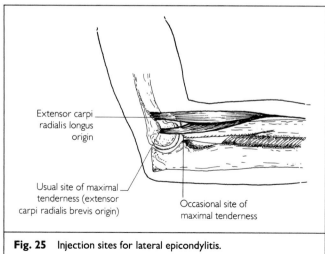

Extensor carpi radialis longus origin

Usual site of maximal tenderness (extensor carpi radialis brevis origin)

Occasional site of maximal tenderness

Fig. 25   Injection sites for lateral epicondylitis.

technique of half-withdrawals and reinsertions. The injection must be made under pressure (the one exception to the rule). Conventionally 1–2 ml is injected, though some prefer larger volumes (2–5 ml) to ensure adequate delivery. Fluorinated steroid should be avoided at this superficial site, the usual choice of injection being hydrocortisone (or methyl prednisolone) in 1% lignocaine. The injection is commonly painful, and the patient should be warned that pain may be exacerbated for 24–48 hours.

Medial epicondylitis ('golfer's elbow')

The situation is very similar to lateral epicondylitis. Position the patient in the same way, and identify the site of maximal tenderness (usually just distal to the medial epicondyle). After warning the patient of probable pain exacerbation, the injection is again made under pressure using a fan technique; a lesser volume of non-fluorinated steroid and lignocaine (1–3 ml) will usually suffice. The ulnar nerve runs behind and below the medial epicondyle and careful siting of the injection is therefore required.

Olecranon bursitis

The bursa is superficial and no important structures traverse its surface. Aspiration is therefore straightforward, the needle being aimed towards the site of maximal distension. Non-fluorinated steroid should be used for injection.

3

THE HAND

Examination of the hand provides information on its function and disease diagnosis. The hand is a complex structure and its examination is a challenge. Since it functions proximal to distal, that is the effective function of its distal parts are dependent on the more proximal components, it is logical that the examination should run from proximal to distal.

Observation is the most important source of information. This starts as the subject walks into the room. The examiner should watch how the hands are used and held, particularly when the patient undresses, and how the patient holds the hands when relaxed. In more detailed examination, the hands should be observed at rest, movement assessed and then specific problems, including examination of peripheral nerves, addressed. By comparing both hands it is frequently easier to identify an abnormality. As problems of the hands are often associated with pathology elsewhere, particularly in the arm and neck, the examination needs to be in the context of a more general assessment.

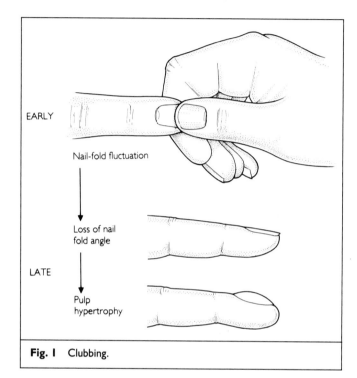

EARLY

Nail-fold fluctuation

Loss of nail fold angle

LATE

Pulp hypertrophy

Fig. I Clubbing.

Examination

Observation needs to be purposeful and should avoid a 'random walk'. It is best done looking proximal to distal following the functional organisation of the hand. Consider the overall aspect of the hand and, in particular, count the digits. It is important to establish that the anatomical configuration is normal with normal longitudinal and lateral arches.

There may be features of specific systemic disease (Figs 1–4). These show as a specific pattern of abnormality, such as clubbing (Fig. 1), cyanosis, leuconychia, splinter haemorrhages or onycholysis. There may be tremor from anxiety, Parkinson's disease or thyrotoxicosis, or a flap from respiratory or liver failure. Signs maybe of an overall change in the hand, such as the large hands and thickened waxy skin of hypothyroidism or the large hands of acromegaly. Deformity with short fat fingers suggests congenital abnormality, achondroplasia, or long thin fingers Marfan's syndrome. In the arthritides the pattern of joint involvement is extremely important in diagnosis (Figs 2–4).

During the examination consider separately the component structures: the skin, muscle, tendons, nerve, bones and joints.

The skin is thicker on the palmar than the dorsal surface. It is tethered to deep structures at the palmar's creases and in the fingers by lateral and medial ligaments (Cleland and Grayson's ligaments). Loss of sweating may indicate nerve damage and there may be evidence of rashes, bruising or solar damage. Eczema characteristically affects the flexures and the palm, whereas a rash from scabies may occur between the fingers. There may be nail change, for example the pitting associated with psoriasis, onycholysis or nail dystrophy. Note any webbing between fingers, and thickening of the skin and fascia. The latter particularly occurs in the lateral aspect of the palm, causing flexion contracture of the fourth and fifth fingers in Dupuytren's contracture (Fig. 5).

Bones and joints

The bones and joints of the hand are organised in a complex array (Fig. 6). Examination allows a number

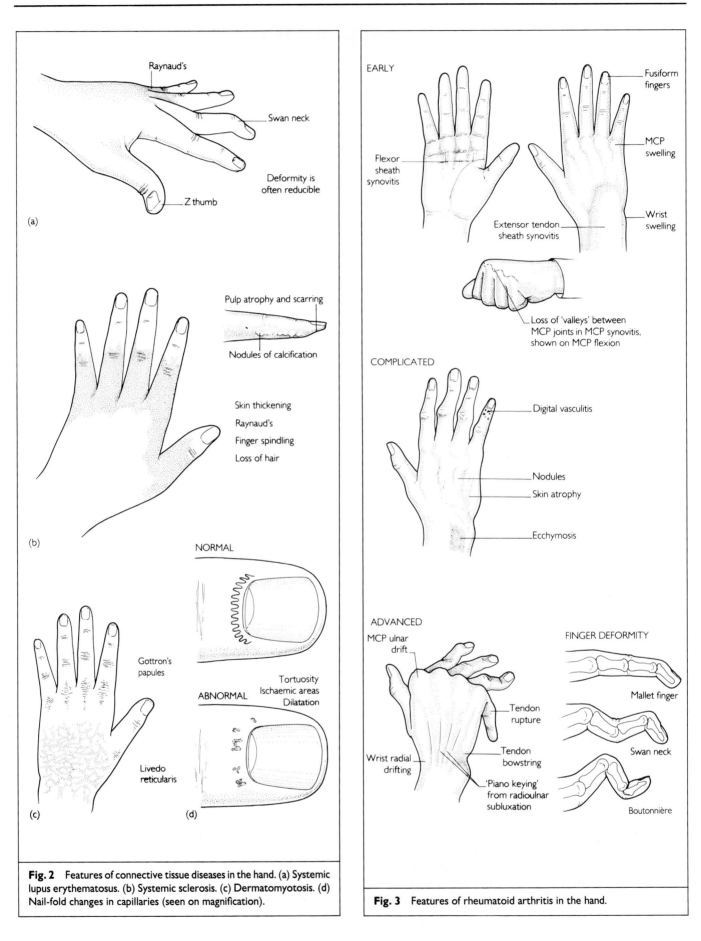

Fig. 2 Features of connective tissue diseases in the hand. (a) Systemic lupus erythematosus. (b) Systemic sclerosis. (c) Dermatomyotosis. (d) Nail-fold changes in capillaries (seen on magnification).

Fig. 3 Features of rheumatoid arthritis in the hand.

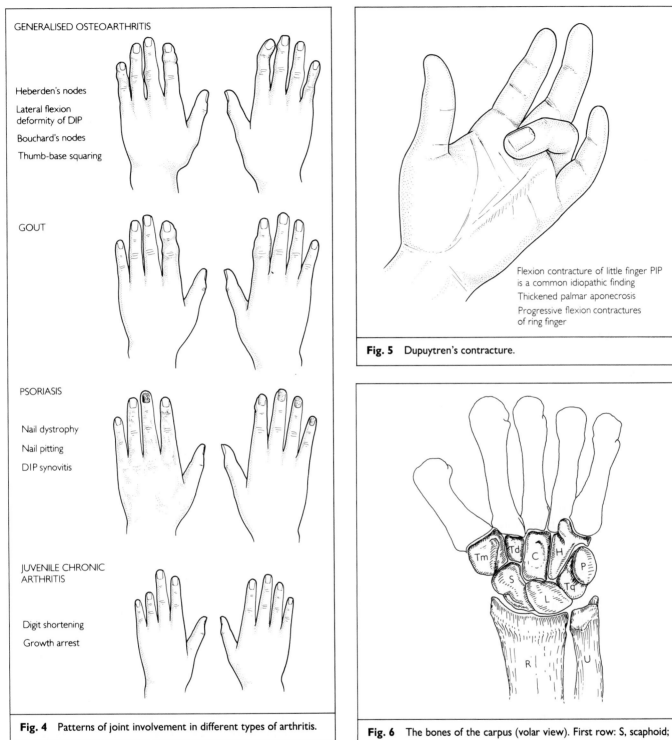

GENERALISED OSTEOARTHRITIS

Heberden's nodes

Lateral flexion
deformity of DIP

Bouchard's nodes

Thumb-base squaring

GOUT

PSORIASIS

Nail dystrophy

Nail pitting

DIP synovitis

**JUVENILE CHRONIC
ARTHRITIS**

Digit shortening

Growth arrest

Fig. 4 Patterns of joint involvement in different types of arthritis.

Flexion contracture of little finger PIP
is a common idiopathic finding
Thickened palmar aponecrosis
Progressive flexion contractures
of ring finger

Fig. 5 Dupuytren's contracture.

Fig. 6 The bones of the carpus (volar view). First row: S, scaphoid; L, lunate; P, pisiform; Tq, triquetrum. Second row: Tm, trapezium; Td, trapezoid; C, capitate; H, hamate. R, Radius; U, ulna.

of features to be defined. On the radial side of the wrist the radial styloid can be felt, and distally the palpating finger will cross the radiocarpal joint, navicular trapezial joint and finally the trapezometacarpal joint at the base of the thumb. The ridge in the middle with the dorsum of the radius (Lister's tubercle) finds a line to the base of the middle finger along which the central joints of the carpus can be felt proximal to distal crossing the radiolunate, lunate capitate and capitate

metacarpal joints. Medial palpation from the ulnar styloid crosses the triquetrium and hamate to the base of the fifth metacarpal. Inferiorly the pisiform and the hook of Hamate can be felt. The latter bounds the canal of Guyon, through which the palmar branch of the median nerve runs. Passive movement of the hand allows the joints and bones to be more easily defined

Table 1. Normal range of joint movement (degrees) in the hand

	Flexion	Extension	Abduction	Adduction
Fingers				
MCPs	90	30–45	20	20*
PIPs	100	0	0	0
DIPs	90	10	0	0
Thumb				
MCP	50	0	70	0
IPJ	90	20	0	0
Wrist	80	70		
(Ulnar deviation 30°, radial 20°)				

* In extension but not in flexion.

to identify localised tenderness. Similarly, palpation along the digits will allow localised tenderness to be identified, and careful assessment in relation to the joint line will identify whether it is periarticular or articular. For example in hypertrophic pulmonary osteodystrophy the distal radius or ulna is tender with periostitis which is less prominent at the joint line. Early symmetrical synovitis of the metacarpophalangeal joints may be first shown by squeezing across the metacarpals to elicit tenderness.

Joint movement (Table 1) is extremely difficult to assess in detail. More important is to identify that the hand can function as a unit. This can be demonstrated by asking the subject to make a fist with their thumb outside. To achieve this the wrist must dorsiflex and the metacarpal and interphalangeal joints flex. Then the patient should be asked to show opposition of the thumb and index and thumb and little finger, and finally asked to spread the hands to show abduction of the fingers and extension of the thumbs. Restriction of movement requires assessment to define whether it is due to tendon or joint problems.

Tendons

Detailed assessment of tendons is complex. It is important to establish whether there is associated tenosynovitis by palpating along the tendon. Palpation of the tendon in tension allows the integrity of the tendon to be fully established and will identify whether there is rupture. The tendons are best considered in groups. The extensor pollicis longus and abductor pollicis longus can be shown as the thumb abducts or is extended. These tendons are frequently involved in tenosynovitis (De Quervain's tenosynovitis). This may cause tenderness associated with the radial styloid. It becomes more prominent by performing Finkelstein's test. The subject is asked to make a fist with the thumb tucked under the fingers and the wrist is then passively flexed and the ulna deviated to stretch the tendon against the radius; this causes pain if the tendon is inflamed.

The extensor carpi radius longus and brevis are assessed by asking the patient first to make a fist and then feeling the tendons under extensor pollicis longus. The extensor pollicis longus runs along the ulnar side of the radial tubercle, turning approximately 45° to the thumb. The extensor indicis and extensor digitorum communis, as well as the extensor digiti minimi, can be observed as the patient flexes the fingers from a clenched fist. The extensor carpi ulnaris can be felt in the groove below the ulnar styloid as the subject deviates the fist in an ulnar direction.

On the palmar aspect of the hand, the palmaris longus becomes prominent when the wrist is flexed at the same time as thumb and little finger oppose. The flexor carpi radialis becomes prominent when the wrist is flexed with the radial deviation. The flexor digitorum sublimis and profundus are assessed by holding the fingers in extension to allow only distal interphalangeal joint flexion from the profundis. If all three fingers apart from the one being examined are held in extension the subject will be able to flex the proximal interphalangeal joint of the free finger if the sublimus tendon to that finger is intact.

The lumbricle muscles arise from the flexor digitorum profundus tendon on the radial side in the palm and pass over the carpometacarpal joints to insert into the lateral slips of the extensor expansion. They therefore flex the metacarpophalangeal and extend the interphalangeal joints.

Muscles

The assessment of the tendons is associated with the assessment of muscle power. The finger extensors are assessed by asking the patient to resist metacarpophalangeal joint extension. Similarly flexion and power can be assessed by asking the patient to make a fist and then resist the observer extending the fingers. Finger adduction is assessed by asking the patient to try to hold a piece of paper between their fingers and the examiner trying to remove it. Finger abduction is assessed by the observer trying to force the extended abducted fingers together. Similarly, power of thumb flexion is established by asking the subject to touch his or her thenar eminence and resist extension, and extension is assessed by asking him or her to extend the thumb against resistance. Abduction is assessed by the subject resisting an attempt to press the thumb back down into the palm; conversely, adduction is assessed by resisting the subject's attempt to adduct the thumb. Opposition strength can be assessed by the patient trying to resist the examiner's attempt to open the 'O ring' created by the opposing thumb and index finger.

The possibility that restricted flexion of the interphalangeal and metacarpophalangeal joint is due to intrinsic muscle disease resulting from lumbricle and interossei shortening rather than to joint disease can be assessed by Bunnel's test. With the metacarpophalangeal joints extended, ask the subject to flex the interphalangeal joints. If flexion is limited, then flex the metacarpophalangeal joints passively. If this allows the interphalangeal joint flexion to increase, there is intrinsic muscle tightness, but if it is unaltered, the interphalangeal joints themselves are the cause of the restriction. Similarly, restriction of the proximal interphalangeal joints may be due either to retinacular restriction or to joint disease. If the subject is asked to extend the proximal interphalangeal joint and flex the distal interphalangeal joints, if flexion of the distal interphalangeal joints is restricted, then flex the proximal interphalangeal joints. The flexion of the proximal interphalangeal joints will allow increased flexion of the distal interphalangeal joint if there is retinacular restriction but not if the restriction is due to joint disease.

Nerves

The analysis of nerve lesions aims to establish whether there is evidence of a neuropathy, mononeuritis of the radial, median or ulnar nerves or of a nerve root entrapment. The dermatone innervation is C6 on the radial aspect, C7 the middle ray of the hand running to the middle finger, with the ulnar aspect from C8. Light touch tested in the lateral aspect of the thumb, the middle finger and medial aspect of the little finger will screen for sensory loss.

Innervation of wrist extensors is root C(6)7 via the radial nerve, and wrist flexion C78 via the median and ulnar nerves. Finger flexion is C8 via the median and ulnar nerve, and extension C8 via the radial nerve. Finger abduction and adduction is T1 root via the ulnar nerve. Loss of power is tested by the subject trying to resist the examiner opposing wrist flexion, wrist extension and finger abduction, and opposition screens the principal root and muscle groups (Fig. 7). Power of a finger adduction is assessed by the subject resisting the examiner pulling a piece of paper from between the fingers (Fig. 8).

The movement of the thumb causes some confusion. As it is rotated compared to the fingers, abduction, adduction and flexion extension are different. The orientation of the thumb-nail provides a plane to orientate correctly (Fig. 9). Weakness of the adductor pollicis is demonstrated by asking the subject to hold a book with the thumb against the index finger (Fig. 10). If the thumb cannot be held extended and flexes at the metacarpal and interphalangeal joints, adductor weakness is present. In the

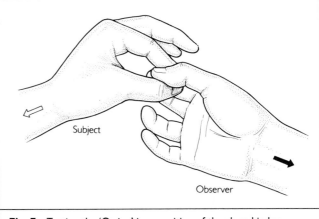

Fig. 7 Testing the 'O ring' in opposition of thumb and index.

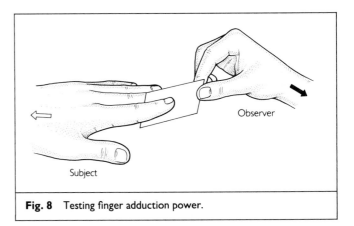

Fig. 8 Testing finger adduction power.

presence of joint signs the neurological or muscle component of weakness is more difficult to assess. Each of the three main peripheral nerves must be assessed (Fig. 11).

The median nerve, (lateral and medial cord of the brachial plexus, C(5)678T1), is characterised by thenar muscle wasting, seen best by comparing hands in a prayer position and by demonstrating weakness of abductor pollicis brevis by resisted abduction of the thumb. Sensory loss in the median nerve area is also common. The common site of entrapment is the carpal tunnel. Symptoms may be severe and gross change be detected on nerve conduction studies even though there may be few signs. Thenar muscle wasting may occur as a result of osteoarthritis of the carpometacarpal joint. The provocation tests of Tinel and Phalen are of limited value in comparison with electrophysiology because of frequent false negatives and false positives. Tinel's sign involves percussing the anterior wrist over the tunnel to induce paraesthesia in the median nerve area. Phalan's sign involves sustained flexion of the wrist for 60 secs, inducing paraesthesia or increased numbness if there is entrapment.

A more proximal lesion of the median nerve above the anterior osseous branch will cause wasting of the

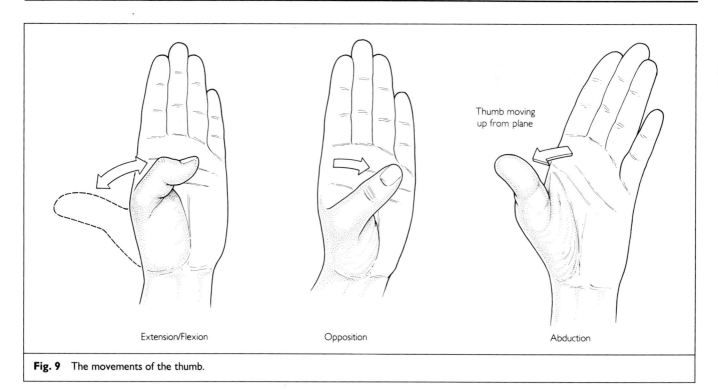

Fig. 9 The movements of the thumb.

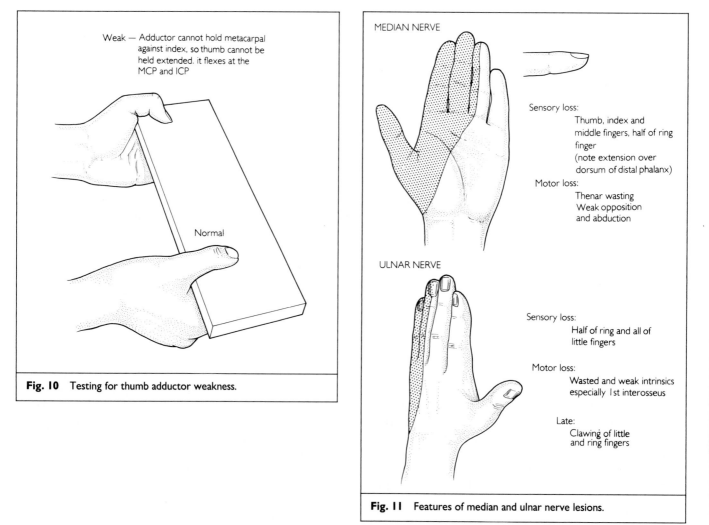

Fig. 10 Testing for thumb adductor weakness.

Fig. 11 Features of median and ulnar nerve lesions.

long flexus, with the index finger being held in extension or the 'Benedictine' attitude. The abductor pollicis brevis is always supplied by the median nerve.

Ulnar nerve (median cord, C8T1), lesions are usually associated with sensory symptoms of loss, and early involvement of the first interosseous muscle is a helpful sign. This is identified by asking the patient to abduct extended fingers. Palpate the dorsal first interosseous. This muscle will also be wasted and weak in a T1 root lesion. The sensory distribution of the nerve supply varies considerably. Occasionally there may be no ulnar cutaneous innervation. Muscle supply is more consistent in the sense that the abductor pollicis brevis is never supplied by the ulna.

An established ulna nerve lesion is characterised by sensory loss and clawing. The metacarpophalangeal joints are extended and the proximophalangeal joints flexed. If the lesion is above the nerve supply to the flexor digitorum profundis the distal interphalangeal joints will be straight, if it is below they will be flexed.

The radial nerve is characterised by weakness of dorsiflexion. If it is mild this may be minimal, but if it is severe there may be profound wrist drop. There would be associated wasting of the muscles of the forearm. Sensory loss, however, may be minimal and confined to a small area on the dorsum of the hand. The level of the nerve entrapment will be indicated by the involvement of the supinator. If this is weak with weak supination established when the arm is extended to counter the effects of the biceps, then the lesion must be proximal to the supinator canal. If it is even more proximal, the triceps may be weak or lost.

Sensory loss may reflect a peripheral neuropathy which will give a characteristic glove pattern. Dissociated sensory loss from posterior column disease or syringomyelia should be examined, particularly if there is small muscle wasting. Sensory loss rarely follows a root pattern. Specific patterns of deformity will result from brachial plexus lesions. In Erb's palsy the wrists and fingers are flexed with extension of the elbow to give the 'Waiter's hands'. This results from involvement of the C5/6 root. In Kumpje's palsy, paralysis of T1 causes a claw hand following intrinsic-muscle paralysis.

Circulation

The circulation of the hand needs to be assessed by checking the presence of the radial and ulnar pulse. Severe hand ischaemia will give specific patterns of deformity (Fig. 12). In Volkmann's contracture, brachial artery occlusion at the elbow will result in forearm wasting with secondary fibrosis causing clawing. Characteristically the fingers may straighten if the wrist is passively flexed. Sensory loss is variable. More distal arterial oclusion may result in Bunnell's contrac-

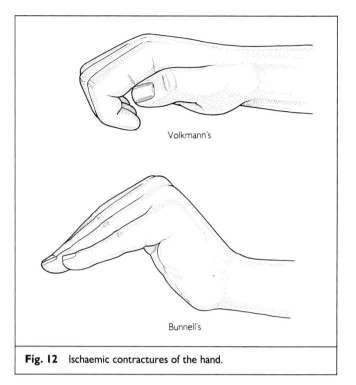

Fig. 12 Ischaemic contractures of the hand.

ture. The metacarpophalangeal joints are flexed with the fingers extended and the thumb adducted.

Satisfactory perfusion of the hand should be sought by demonstrating the presence of a radial artery. The pattern of perfusion can be illustrated by asking the subject to squeeze the hand after first occluding the ulnar and radial artery with firm finger pressure. The release of one will result in a flush to the perfusion area.

Deformity

Observation of the hands at rest will identify deformity. Observe them proximal to distal. Dorsally there may be wrist and radial subluxation and prominence of the ulnar styloid due to subluxation of the radial ulnar joint. There may be small-muscle wasting of the intrinsics. Collapse of the carpus and wrist subluxation will cause bowstring of the extensor tendons and give apparent wasting. Swellings should be defined in association with the surrounding anatomy, for example the extent of tendon sheath synovitis on the dorsum of the hand restricted by the extensor retinaculum. There may be thenar muscle wasting and thumb-base squaring. The palmar aponeurosis may be thickened from Dupuytren's contracture.

A number of deformities of the fingers are characteristic. The rupture of the distal slip of the extensor expansion results in a mallet finger. Heberden's nodes form around the distal interphalangeal joint from osteoarthritis. Proximal interphalangeal joint

osteoarthritis causes bony swelling termed Bouchard's nodes. Hyperextension of the proximal interphalangeal joint gives a swan neck deformity. Flexion
of the proximal interphalangeal joint and extension of
the distal interphalangeal joint gives the boutonnière
deformity (Fig. 3).

Examination of the Acutely Traumatised Hand

Examination in an emergency takes a different per-
spective. Time is important and the identification of
problems requiring immediate action are a priority. In
particular, the adequacy of blood supply is vital. It is
important to carefully document traumatic lesions and
to recognise that, as the injury evolves, more detailed
assessment may be required later.

Screening Examination of the Hand

Look at both hands dorsally when they are resting.
Look proximal to distally. Then ask the patient to turn
his or her hands over to show the palm surface.
Observe a power grip, thumb outside and a pinch
grip. Feel the pulse and feel for tenderness. Test touch
sensation on the lateral aspect of the little finger's
dorsum or the medial aspect of the index finger. Test
for power of the first dorsal interosseous and the
abductor pollicis brevis.

Injection

Steroid injection is effective in reducing the swelling
and pain associated with joint and tendon sheath
inflammation. Possibly because it reduces tendon
sheath swelling, injection may be effective in reducing
the symptoms of carpal tunnel syndrome.

The cardinal principles of local steroid injection
therapy are the same principles as described for other
sites.

Avoid the potential hazard of an intensely catabolic
drug causing tissue damage that may result in nerve
damage or tendon rupture.

- It is essential to be familiar with the local anatomy.
- Check the needle is correctly placed.
- Never inject against resistance.

Carpal tunnel

The nerve runs superficially in close approximation to
flexor pollicis longus and flexor digitorum super-

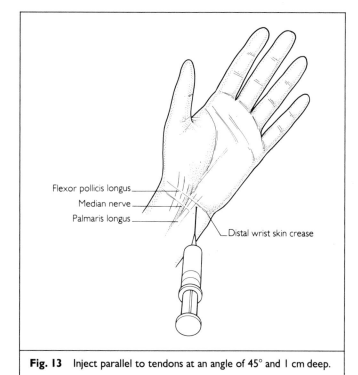

Fig. 13   Inject parallel to tendons at an angle of 45° and 1 cm deep.

ficialis. These tendons can be identified by asking the
patient to flex the wrist. Insert a fine-gauge needle into
the tunnel at an angle 45° and 1 cm deep into the distal
palmar crease which is just medial to the palmaris
tendon (Fig. 13). Check that the needle is not in a
tendon by asking the subject to flex and extend their
fingers and then inject 5–10 mg Triamcinolone or
equivalent. Ensure that there is no resistance to injection and that there is no pain or paraesthesia in the
median nerve distribution.

Flexor sheaths

Insert a fine-gauge needle into a flexor sheath, which
just proximal to the metacarpal crease, laterally along
the tendon (Fig 14). Check that the needle has been
correctly inserted by asking the subject to flex the
finger to show only a minimal movement of the
needle. Then reattach the syringe and inject 5 mg
Triamcinolone or equivalent into the flexor sheath,
withdrawing the needle as this is done.

Metacarpal and interphalangeal joints (Fig. 15)

The joint line should be identified by gently flexing
and extending the joint (note it is more proximal than
the bend of the flexed finger would suggest). Using
the superolateral approach ensure that the neurovascular bundle has been avoided and then inject. The
patient should feel the joint being expanded. Use no
more than 5 mg Triamcinolone.

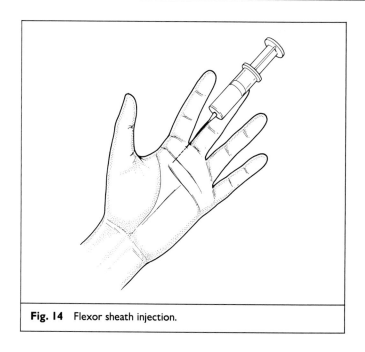

Fig. 14 Flexor sheath injection.

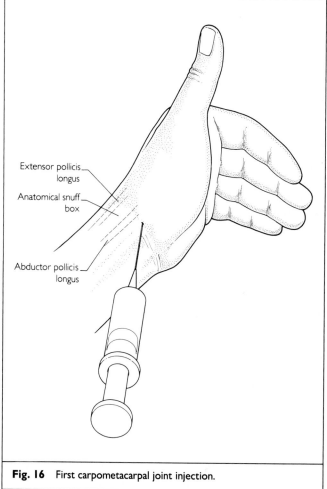

Extensor pollicis longus

Anatomical snuff box

Abductor pollicis longus

Fig. 16 First carpometacarpal joint injection.

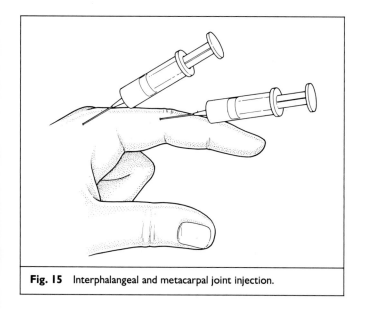

Fig. 15 Interphalangeal and metacarpal joint injection.

be identified by palpation and the injection is carried out whilst holding the wrist in a partially flexed position. Inject using a superior approach to the joint space just medial to the ulnar styloid, or lateral to the extensor pollicis longus tendon. Use 20 mg Triamcinolone or equivalent.

First carpometacarpal joint

The pain of osteoarthritis is the main indication for local injection of this joint. In osteoarthritis there is likely to be extensive osteophyte and thickening of the capsule which makes the insertion of a needle difficult. The joint line should be identified by palpation. Then inject from the lateral aspect near the abductor tendon (Fig. 16). Use 5–7.5 mg Triamcinolone.

Wrist (Fig. 17)

Usually injection is done into the radiocarpal joints or just distal to the ulnar styloid. The joint space should

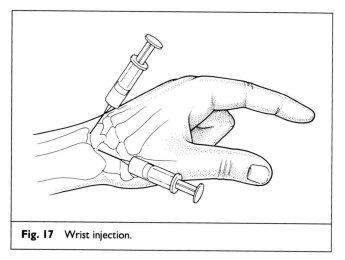

Fig. 17 Wrist injection.

4

THE SPINE

Examination of the spine should establish whether function is impaired and provide evidence of possible underlying disease. Though the spine is a unit, its examination is only part of the wider examination of the locomotor system. Moreover, the close juxtaposition of the neck, thorax and abdomen means that examination must be supported by wider physical assessment and be in the context of the clinical history.

The spine has six major functions. It acts as a scaffold from which the structures of the chest and abdomen are hung. These structures in turn stabilise the spine. It acts as a crane allowing bending and upper-limb lifting. It acts to position the upper limbs and head. It acts as a base from which movement of the ribs, the arms and the legs can be organised. It acts as a protective channel for the spinal cord. It acts as a vibration damper, with low energy absorbed out by the discs and muscles, avoiding continuous vibration injury to the brain during movement.

These functions create conflicting demands between movement and stability. This is resolved by the spine's organisation in small units as an array of vertebrae. Each unit can move a small amount, and that small deflection can be stabilised. The sum of these movements allows the necessary large deflection (Fig. 1).

The unit is composed of a vertebral body with its body and neural arch. The vertebra is stacked with interposed vertebral discs. The second posterior column is composed of the vertebral arches linked by synovial apophyseal joints. There are seven cervical, 12 thoracic, five lumbar and five sacral vertebrae. The coccygeal vertebrae are vestigial and the sacral ones fused to form the single sacral bones. The array is organised in three curves: cervical lordosis, thoracic kyphosis and lumbar lordosis.

Development

The spine forms as a result of the condensation of mesanchyme after formation of the primitive streak in the embryonal disc. The formation of the notochord parallels the formation of the neural tube. Tissue then segments to form a series of myotomes, sclerotomes and dermatomes. Subsequent fusion of the sacral vertebrae creates the single sacral bones. Frequently at the lumbar sacral junction there may be various combinations of fusions of the transverse processes and vertebrae. This may result in sacralisation of L5 as it fuses to the sacrum, or failure of fusion of S1-determined lumbarisation of S1. Incomplete formation of the spinal canal results in spina bifida. Diseases affecting the spine before skeletal maturity and epyphiseal fusion will produce defects which are compounded by growth.

The embryogenesis of the neck is particularly complex. After formation of the phalangeal arches there is relative migration of structures. So, for example, the diaphragm from the C5 myotome moves caudally. The migration of structures produces relationships that determine the pattern of referred pain. It may also result in lost or vestigial structures that fail to satisfactorily migrate. Because the upper limb is produced from the elongation of the C5 to T1 segments, pain from the neck may be referred to the arm.

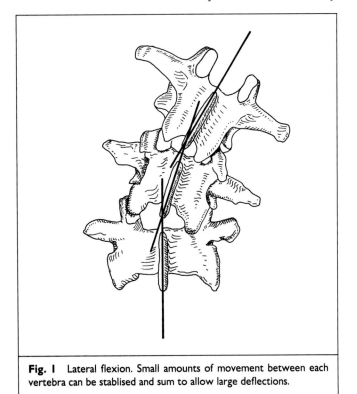

Fig. 1 Lateral flexion. Small amounts of movement between each vertebra can be stablised and sum to allow large deflections.

THE CERVICAL SPINE

The cervical spine is examined in conjunction with an examination of the neck. In addition, as so many structures pass through the cervical spine, the impact of problems may be found distally. In particular, disease affecting the cervical cord or roots may produce neurological abnormality in the arms or legs.

Functional Anatomy

In the mature skeleton the intervetebral discs do not completely cover the vertebral plate, so laterally two synovial joints develop; the uncovertebral joints. The vertebral artery ascends in close association to the posterior column through the lateral foramina. The upper two vertebrae are specifically modified, with the 'body' of the atlas becoming the dens of the axis. The anterior column is close to the posterior wall of the pharynx. The vertebral canal is relatively narrow at the root of the neck and widens superiorly. Moreover, the cord is expanded in its lower section. This means that canals with a sagittal diameter of less than 13 mm are vulnerable to cord compression (the normal sagittal diameter is between 15 and 20 mm). In flexion, the cord must stretch approximately 2 cm and tends to buckle in extension. Its movement is limited by nerve roots and the ligamentum denticulatum laterally. The cervical nerve roots emerge superior to their respective vertebral bodies. So, for example, C6 root emerges above the vertebral body of C6 and is therefore approximated to the C5/6 discs. The roots input into the brachial plexus from which fibres interchange into the peripheral nerves of the upper limb.

A complete set of muscles provide power for movement. The muscles can be considered in layers and essentially are a superficial sheet of muscles including the trapezius and a deeper band of intrinsic muscles, including long muscles and intrinsic muscles between spinous processes. The resultant movement of the components of the neck allow flexion/extension in the sagittal plane as well as lateral flexion and rotation. To achieve rotation, an element of lateral flexion is necessary. The atlanto-occipital and atlanto-axial component of the spine is particularly mobile. The atlanto-occipital joint accounts for approximately 20° of flexion and 5° of lateral flexion. Rotation is minimal. However at the atlanto-axial joint there is 15° of rotation. Maximal rotation is achieved with some extension and lateral flexion to slacken the alar ligaments.

Movement of each component of the lower cervical spine produces a resultant flexion/extension of 110°, that is flexion from 0 to 85° and extension from 0 to 15°. It is limited by soft-tissue structure. Lateral flexion of 40° and axial rotation of 50° is possible to each side. With age there is a gradual reduction of range of movement. Nodding is a movement largely occurring at the atlanto-occipital joints. The muscles brought into play to achieve any particular movement depend considerably on whether the neck is vertical or supine.

Examination

Much of the examination of the neck is dependent on observation. This begins as soon as the subject walks into the room and is revealed by how the subject holds the neck as he or she sits down. If the whole spine is being examined it may be easiest to examine the neck with the patient standing. It is necessary, in addition, to examine the neck when the patient is lying, when the muscles are relaxed. It may also be necessary to examine associated structures, in particular the ear, the temporomandibular joint and pharynx. Observe the neck anteriorly, laterally and posteriorly.

Anterior observation (Fig. 2) should establish whether the neck is held straight with both shoulders level and eyes level, or if there is a torticollis. A prominent thyroid may be identified and filling of the sternoclavicular angle, possibly with a sternoclavicular lymphadenopathy, may be seen.

Laterally the normal contour of the neck with a cervical lordosis on the thoracic kyphosis should be observed (Fig. 2). If there is a marked thoracic kyphosis this may in turn produce a compensatory hyperextension of the neck. Posteriorly, again examine for deformity and note the particular prominence of the spinous processes of T1, and to a lesser extent C7. A number of specific deformities may be apparent such as a short rigid neck, possibly following Kippel–Feil deformity or resulting from juvenile chronic arthritis. A webbed neck is associated with Turner's syndrome. In infancy, torticollis may be associated with a sternocleidomastoid tumour. In adults it is often secondary to disc disease, scarring, trauma or strabismus.

Palpation will allow the character of the deformity to be analysed. It is important to establish whether there is localised tenderness. Gentle percussion over the vertebra may identify focal tenderness. Lymph nodes should be palpated along the sternocleidomastoid, the occipital line and in the supraclavicular fossi. Similarly, the submandibular and the parotid glands should be felt. The thyroid may be palpable and may be more easily felt if the patient simultaneously swallows some water. This is best done with a person sitting and the examiner feeling from behind, having re-assured the patient that they are not about to be

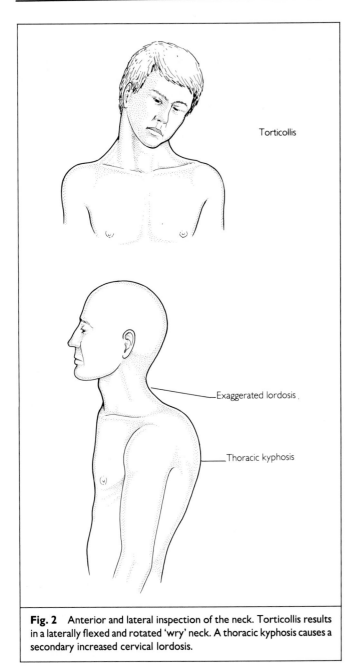

Fig. 2 Anterior and lateral inspection of the neck. Torticollis results in a laterally flexed and rotated 'wry' neck. A thoracic kyphosis causes a secondary increased cervical lordosis.

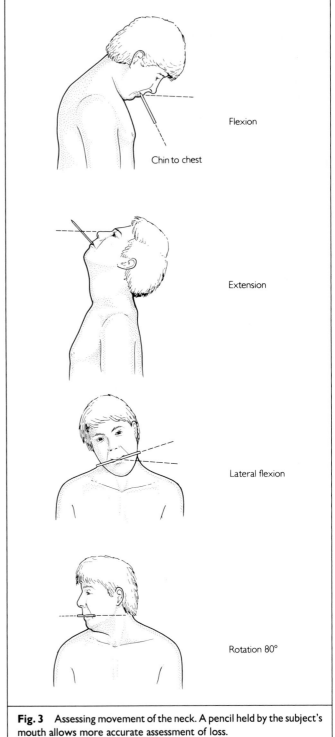

Fig. 3 Assessing movement of the neck. A pencil held by the subject's mouth allows more accurate assessment of loss.

strangled! The thyroid may also be palpated with the patient relaxed as supine. Both carotid pulses should be identified and, if vascular disease is suspected, auscultate for possible bruits.

The neck can then be examined to assess movement (Fig. 3). This is easiest done with the patient seated or standing. It is important to explain the movement being assessed; if necessary, the examiner should demonstrate it. Frequently the subjects are asked to put their ear to their shoulder and will bring their shoulder up to their ear, demonstrating shoulder movement rather than neck movement. The pattern of movement is also important. Is it smooth or jerky and restricted as a result of pain?

The extent of movement is difficult to document but more precise measurement can be achieved by asking the patient to hold a pencil in his or her mouth. Held laterally this allows rotation and lateral flexion to be judged. Held forward, it allows flexion extension to be measured. As a 'rule of thumb', 10° of flexion restriction means that one finger can be placed between the chin and chest wall, and each additional finger implies a further 10° loss. In full extension, the tip of the nose and the forehead should form a horizontal line and the occiput will rotate to the level of the first thoracic spine. In rotation, the chin should turn almost to the shoulder in the coronal line. If the head is gently held during active movement and the range of movement restricted, further pressure can establish whether the range can be increased passively and whether this is painful. If there is any risk of cervical cord damage, this manœuvre should not be performed.

Because of the complexity of the array of muscles in the neck it is impossible to assess individual muscle groups, though there are two exceptions. The trapezius which has an action shrugging the shoulders can be assessed against the resistance of the examiner's hands pushing down. The sternocleidomastoids can be assessed by rotating the neck against resistance and the examiner palpating the contracting muscles. Their action demonstrates the integrity of the eleventh cranial nerve. The power of the flexors can be assessed by asking the patient when lying to put his or her chin on the chest. This can be resisted with a hand on the forehead. The extensors' power can be assessed by the examiner placing a hand on the occiput and assess resistance to extension. Lateral flexion can be assessed by one of the examiner's hands restricting the movement of the shoulder whilst the other resists the laterally flexing head. For rotation, one hand can resist rotation by holding the mandible whilst the other restricts the movement of the shoulder. The ability of a patient to hold the neck flexed for a minute is a screen for muscle power loss and for problems with muscle fatigue, as may occur in polymyositis or myasthenia.

A number of specific tests help clarify particular diagnostic problems. Flexion of the neck may produce paraesthesia in the arms or legs due to nerve irritation. This occurs in cervical spondylosis and multiple sclerosis and is described as the *Barber's chair* or *Lhermitte's* sign. Downward pressure on the head may induce symptoms from vertebral foramina narrowing, particularly if the head is laterally flexed to the side of the expected narrowing. Pressure for 10 secs should induce root pain, but this should not be done if there is any risk of fracture, metastatic lesion or odontoid disease. This is termed *Spurling's manœuvre*. Conver-

sely, cervical traction, by pulling the neck cranially with one hand under the jaw and the second under the occiput, may relieve the symptoms of a compressed root. Pain in a dermatome distribution may be induced from the *Valsalva manœuvre*. Holding the breath against a closed glottis or coughing increases the interthecal pressure and may induce pain from a disc or interthecal tumour.

A number of manœuvres have been advocated for assessing thoracic outlet problems. They aim to increase the obstruction of the lower brachial plexus and to increase restriction to the subclavian arteries. This should result in paraesthesia in the lower cervical roots dermatomes or the loss of the radial pulse combined with a bruit in the clavicular region. One procedure is to raise the arm, extended and externally rotated, to rotate the head towards the arm and take a deep breath. This is one of the many procedures described as *Adson's manœuvre*. However, there is considerable controversy as to both the specificity and sensitivity of the manœuvre in defining significant thoracic outlet problems. Pulling the arm down against the trunk may also reduce pulse-volume change from a possible thoracic outlet obstruction.

Localisation of neurological abnormality in the neck requires a formal neurological examination both of the upper and lower limbs. With nerve root entrapment, symptoms poorly localise to a dermatome. However, a reflex loss may give a level of a lesion, particularly if associated with distal long track signs and increased tone and hyperreflexia. Cervical myelopathy may primarily present with symptoms and signs in the legs. With atlanto-axial subluxation, disturbance to the hind brain, and in particular to arterial supply, may produce a complex pattern involving cranial nerves in addition to abnormalities in the peripheral neurological system. A similar complex pattern may result from intrinsic cord lesions following syringomyelia and the Brown–Sequard syndrome. Similarly, brachial plexus lesions will produce a specific neurological pattern. C5/6 damage results in Erbe's palsy. C8/T1 lower brachial plexus root lesion results in Klumje's deformity. Finally, damage to the sympathetic trunk will give an autonomic problem and may cause Horner's syndrome.

THE THORACIC SPINE

In contrast to the cervical and lumbar spine, the thoracic has restricted mobility and much greater stability. The stability results from the buttressing effects of the thoracic cage. Each vertebra has two sets of three articulations for the ribs. Movement of the rib is an important component of respiration: contraction of

the extrinsic intercostals raises the ribs in inspiration and the diaphragm contracts to flatten at the same time. The anterior abdominal muscles also contract. In expiration, the internal intercostal muscles contract; coordinated with contraction of transverse abdominis and thoracis as well as the subcostals, this depresses the ribs. Examination primarily identifies whether there is a deformity. Movement is much more difficult to assess precisely.

Examination

When observed from the side (Fig. 4) the normal configuration of the thoracic kyphosis can be seen. This may be increased, with a general increase in the curve or with a local acute increase such as occurs in a gibbus, which may result from infection, or fracture. A more gradual increase in the curve occurs in a spondarthritis such as ankylosing spondylitis, Scheurmann's disease, degenerative disc disease, osteoporosis, polio or muscular dystrophy. There may be an associated compensatory cervical hyperextension. A marked thoracic kyphosis will result in abdominal cramping and cause folding of the cramped abdominal wall.

Examination of the thoracic spine from behind allows assessment of whether it is straight or whether there is an element of a scoliosis (Fig. 5). This is a lateral bend. A small degree of scoliosis is a frequently observed normal feature. However, pronounced scoliosis needs full assessment. A scoliosis may be compensatory, postural or fixed. A compensatory scoliosis results from leg-length inequality. This can be identified by examining the patient sitting, when postural scoliosis should be abolished. Then the leg

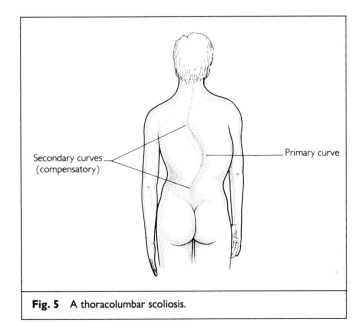

Fig. 5 A thoracolumbar scoliosis.

Secondary curves (compensatory)

Primary curve

should be assessed for relative shortening. If when sitting the scoliosis persists, ask the patient to bend forward. If the curve disappears, this suggests the scoliosis is mobile and it is most likely that it is postural in origin. If it persists, it suggests a structural fixed scoliosis, which should become more pronounced. The associated deformity of the chest wall produces a rib hump. This is because not only is the spine laterally flexed but it is also rotated. The body of the vertebra rotates to the convexity and the spinous process to the concavity of the curve. There are usually three curves. The middle one is primary and fixed, the one or two compensatory curves above and below may then become fixed later. Once the deformity has developed, it is likely to increase because of growth effects. The primary curve is described to indicate whether the scoliosis is convex to the left or to the right. Commonly scoliosis is idiopathic. However, it is important to explore the possibility that it is secondary to neurological disease, in particular polio, neurofibromatosis, syringomyelia or a myopathy. It may be congenital, secondary to abnormalities such as fused hemivertebra or absent discs. It also may be as a result of focal inflammation or neoplasm. In particular, the latter may be associated with pain, and it is extremely important to investigate a possible secondary cause if there is associated tenderness or pain.

There are five main patterns of idiopathic scoliosis. In *infantile thoracic scolioses*, 90% are convex to the left and 60% occur in males. In *adolescent thoracic kyphoses*, 90% occur in females and 90% are convex to the right, over 50% develop a severe scoliosis. A *thoracolumbar scoliosis* is more common in females and slightly more common to the right. A *lumbar scoliosis* is more common in females, it occurs equally to the right or

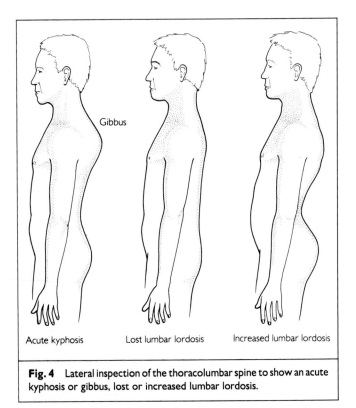

Gibbus

Acute kyphosis   Lost lumbar lordosis   Increased lumbar lordosis

Fig. 4 Lateral inspection of the thoracolumbar spine to show an acute kyphosis or gibbus, lost or increased lumbar lordosis.

left, it is not associated with a thoracic cage abnormality and is therefore frequently missed until it presents as backache in adult life. *Thoracic and lumbar scolioses* may be combined to produce a compensatory curve and relatively little deformity.

A kyphosis and scoliosis will restrict chest wall movement and consequently will frequently be associated with respiratory problems. Examination of the thoracic spine should therefore be combined with an examination of the respiratory system.

Movement of the thoracic spine is best assessed by noting the increased distance between D1 and D12 in anterior flexion. This should normally be at least 3 cm. This represents 45° of flexion. Approximately 20° of extension may also occur. Lateral flexion is best assessed by observing from behind and watching the spine move as the patient runs one hand down one

side of his or her leg. The average range of movement is 15° to either side. Flexion, extension and lateral flexion are integrated with lumbar spine movement, so limitation of movement needs to be carefully assessed against what is expected overall for the thoracolumbar spine. Rotation may be assessed by fixing the pelvis, easiest done by asking the patient to sit and then asking him or her to twist to look over the shoulder. Thoracic movement is approximately 35° and is added to by a much more limited 5° of lumbar rotation. Finally movement of the costovertebral joints can be assessed by the amount of chest expansion, normally measured at the 'nipple line'. This should be more than 5 cm. Finally, focal tenderness in the thoracic spine should be assessed by gently percussing the thoracic vertebrae.

THE LUMBAR SPINE

Examination of the lumbar spine is frequently combined with examination of the thoracic spine. Observation will allow the identification of deformities. In particular, observed laterally, a loss of the normal lumbar lordosis may frequently occur secondary to disc disease. The lordosis may be increased as a result of a spondylolisthesis, fixed flexion deformity of the hips, obesity, pregnancy and poor posture. Examining from behind will allow the straightness of the spine to be assessed and scoliosis to be identified. This frequently is secondary to degenerative disc and apophyseal disease.

The smoothness of movement and restriction of movement is assessed examining the patient from the side and from behind. Anterior flexion should result in an increase in the distance between D12 and S1 of greater than 7 cm. The distance of the tips of the extended fingers to the floor gives an index of combined hip and spinal flexion, and should normally be less than 10 cm. However, hip flexion can compensate to a considerable extent for loss of spinal flexion. Hypermobility is associated with increased flexion and extension to the point where the person may be able to put the hands flat on the floor. Lateral flexion occurs to approximately 15° on either side in the lumbar spine, rotation occurs to approximately 5° to either side.

Spinal disease is frequently associated with abdominal problems (Fig. 6). A full abdominal assessment is therefore necessary in addition. In particular, the possible presence of a psoas abscess presenting as an inguinal mass should be explored. Vaginal examination may be appropriate. Frequently, lumbar spine problems are associated with nerve root entrapment, which needs specific assessment.

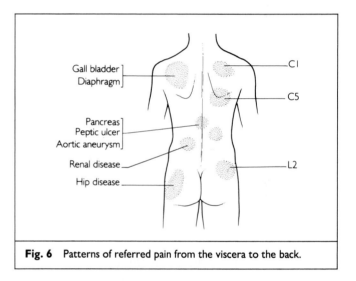

Fig. 6 Patterns of referred pain from the viscera to the back.

Pain due to root entrapment may be analysed by specific measures to assess root irritation (Fig. 7). It may also be necessary to perform tests to clarify whether a patient is malingering.

The femoral nerve roots L2, 3 and 4, may be stressed by asking the patient to lie prone, then flexing the knee to cause mild pain, which is exacerbated when the hip is extended.

Sciatic nerve roots L4 and 5, S1, 2 and 3 may be stressed with a number of measures. With the patient supine, flex the hip with a straight leg. Normally this can be done to 90°. Limitation of flexion before the fault is achieved, in the presence of a normal hip, suggests root disease. Flex the knee to allow further flexion of the hip and then straighten the knee to see if this induces pain (*Lasegue test*). If it does, confirm root irritation by easing knee flexion to what is tolerable

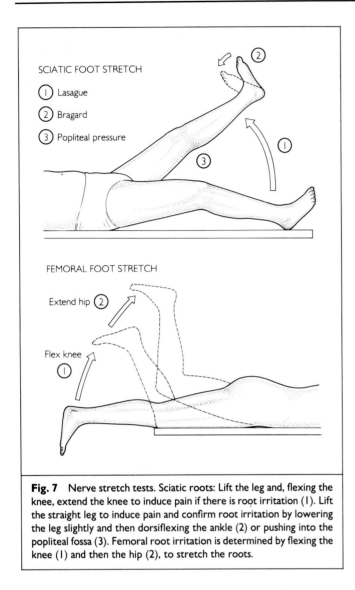

SCIATIC FOOT STRETCH
① Lasague
② Bragard
③ Popliteal pressure

FEMORAL FOOT STRETCH

Extend hip ②

Flex knee ①

Fig. 7   Nerve stretch tests. Sciatic roots: Lift the leg and, flexing the knee, extend the knee to induce pain if there is root irritation (1). Lift the straight leg to induce pain and confirm root irritation by lowering the leg slightly and then dorsiflexing the ankle (2) or pushing into the popliteal fossa (3). Femoral root irritation is determined by flexing the knee (1) and then the hip (2), to stretch the roots.

and then dorsiflex the ankle (*Bragard test*). Finally, increased pressure in the popliteal fossa may induce root irritation (*bowstring test*). Following this, ask the patient to sit up and observe that, if there is root irritation, he or she should flex the knees to ease root pressure as they sit up. Malingering or 'functional overlay' may be suggested by inconsistency in the pattern of signs. The pain may be worse compressing the spine by pressing on the head or illiciting peripheral pain with a pinch. One common inconsistency will be determined by the amount of rotation of the spine required to induce pain. If the patient is standing and asked to rotate the shoulders with hands free, the rotation will primarily be spinal. If the patient is then asked to hold the hands by his or her side and rotate the spine again, pain induced at the same position is very strongly suggestive of a functional cause, as the predominant movement should be occurring in the legs.

The pattern of pain in the lower limbs gives an

indication of the probable level of a nerve lesion. The hard signs however are the loss of a reflex, supported by muscle weakness and possibly wasting. An L4 root lesion will be associated with the loss of the knee reflex and weakness of the quadriceps, an L5 root with weakness of the extensor hallucis longus, and an S1 root with the loss of the ankle reflex and weakness of the soleus.

The cord ends at the level of the L2 vertebra in the adult. A central disc protrusion at this level or above will cause a paraparesis; below this level neurological disease or extrinsic compression will produce a syndrome of multiple root involvement. This is termed the cauda equina syndrome (Fig. 8). There are primarily two patterns. A high lateral lesion will result in root lesions with lower parametal signs. A midline (conus) lesion will give saddle sensory loss but frequently no motor loss until the S1 root results in ankle weakness.

A spondylolisthesis may show no deformity and present primarily with nerve and cord entrapment. A transverse lumbar crease and a palpable step in the lumbar spine are weak signs that can heighten suspicion of a problem that requires detailed neurological examination. Similarly, spinal stenosis may be suspected from the history; it is important to establish whether it is associated with peripheral vascular disease in the lower limbs.

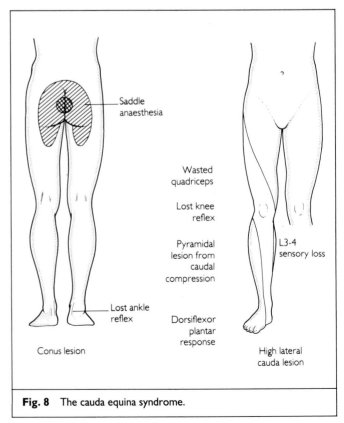

Saddle anaesthesia

Wasted quadriceps

Lost knee reflex

Pyramidal lesion from caudal compression

Lost ankle reflex

L3-4 sensory loss

Dorsiflexor plantar response

Conus lesion

High lateral cauda lesion

Fig. 8   The cauda equina syndrome.

The Sacroiliac Joints

The sacroiliac joints are extremely difficult to assess. They have minimal movement and probably only limited information could be derived about local tenderness (Fig. 9). Pain may be induced by trying to compress the pelvis or by distracting it and pushing it across the iliac blades. A similar destruction procedure flexing the hip and knee and forcibly adducting the leg across to the contralateral iliac fossa may also induce pain. However, the specificity of these tests is likely to be poor, with many false positives.

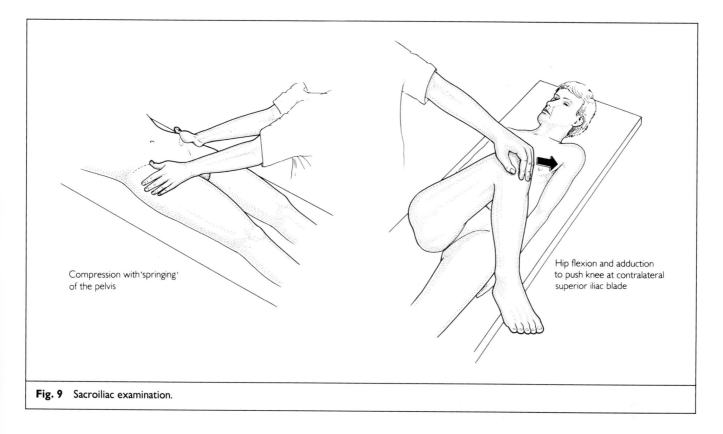

Compression with 'springing' of the pelvis

Hip flexion and adduction to push knee at contralateral superior iliac blade

Fig. 9   Sacroiliac examination.

5

THE HIP

The hip is a synovium-lined ball-and-socket joint that combines an extensive range of movement with great stability. The stability is due to the relatively deep insertion of the femoral head into the acetabulum and the strong capsule and muscles that surround the joint. The hip plays a major role in weight-bearing and locomotion, so that disorders of the hip are translated quickly into pain and limp. Disordered hip function also disturbs sexual activity.

Development

The lower limb buds appear at approximately 4 weeks of embryonic life as small lateral outgrowths of the trunk opposite the lumbar and upper sacral segments. At birth, the acetabulum is entirely cartilaginous and sited at the meeting point of the ilium, pubis and ischium which, at this stage of development, are the three separate centres making up the hemipelvis. The centre of ossification in the head of the femur is visible on X-ray at 6 months, while the centre of ossification appears in the greater trochanter at approximately 7 years of age. In adolescence, the head of the femur is well-developed and three epiphyseal lines can be seen: between the head and neck of the femur and outlining the greater and lesser trochanters. These begin to fuse shortly after puberty and fusion is usually complete by the age of 20 years.

Developmental abnormalities

Congenital dislocation of the hip affects approximately 1 in 1000 babies. One or both hips may be dislocated at birth or dislocate in the first few weeks of life. Girls are affected more than boys and there is a familial tendency. All neonates should be routinely examined for this. The condition can be detected by flexing the hips and knees (Fig. 1) and abducting the hips. Normally, the thigh will touch or nearly touch the examining couch. If there is subluxation of the hip, abduction will be limited. The femoral head may be felt slipping into the acetabulum, sometimes with an audible click.

The blood supply to the epiphysis of the head of the femur is vulnerable between the ages of 5 and 10 years.

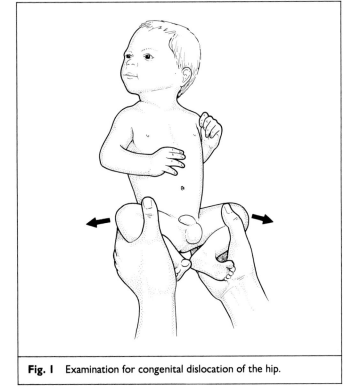

Fig. I Examination for congenital dislocation of the hip.

In Perthes' disease, blood supply is impaired, leading to osteonecrosis of the capital epiphysis and resulting in a flattened, misshapen head of the femur.

Slipped femoral epiphysis is a disorder of adolescence affecting boys more than girls. The head of the femur slips inferiorly and posteriorly on the neck, leading to a coxa vara deformity of the hip. This can occur acutely or, more commonly, as a subacute process. Sometimes there is a history of trauma, but mostly the cause is unknown.

Contraction of the iliotibial band can result in a deformity consisting of flexion, abduction and external rotation of the hip, unequal leg length, pelvic tilt and exaggerated lumbar lordosis, valgus deformity and flexion contracture of the knee, external torsion of the tibia on the femur and a secondary equinovarus deformity of the foot. Partial forms of this are most commonly encountered and it is an important cause, for example, of instability of the knee.

Anatomy

The proximal part of the femur (Fig. 2) consists of the head, neck, and greater and lesser trochanters which are joined by the intertrochanteric line. The head articulates in the acetabular cavity, which is deepened by the glenoid labrum, a circular fibrocartilaginous rim that forms a tight collar around the head of the femur. A gap in the lower portion of the labrum, the acetabular notch, is bridged by the transverse ligament, beneath which blood vessels pass into the joint. The articular cartilage of the acetabulum is horseshoe-shaped, and a mass of fat lies in the fossa at the bottom of the acetabulum.

There is a strong, dense fibrous capsule. This is attached proximally to the acetabulum, the glenoid facet and the transverse ligament. Distally, it covers the lateral margin of the femoral head and most of the neck. Anteriorly it is attached to the intertrochanteric line and posteriorly to the neck just above this (Fig. 2). The capsule is reinforced in front by the iliofemoral ligament, inferiorly by the pubofemoral ligament and behind by the ischiofemoral ligament.

The ligamentum teres is an intracapsular ligament which arises from the transverse ligament of the acetabular rim, attaching to a pit in the head of the femur, and carries blood vessels which provide nourishment for a small area of the head adjacent to the attachment of the ligament. On the inner aspect of the distal part of the capsule, fibrous bands carry blood vessels to foramina of the neck and femoral head.

The iliotibial band is a portion of the fascia lata. It extends down the lateral thigh from its major attachment at the iliac crest to the lateral tibial tubercle.

The synovial membrane lines the inner surface of the articular capsule. It covers the glenoid labrum and the mass of fat in the bottom of the acetabular cavity. It also encloses the ligamentum teres. Distally, it is reflected onto the femoral neck and extends to the articular cartilage of the head (Fig. 2).

Many bursae have been identified. Those most involved clinically are the iliopectineal bursa, the tro-

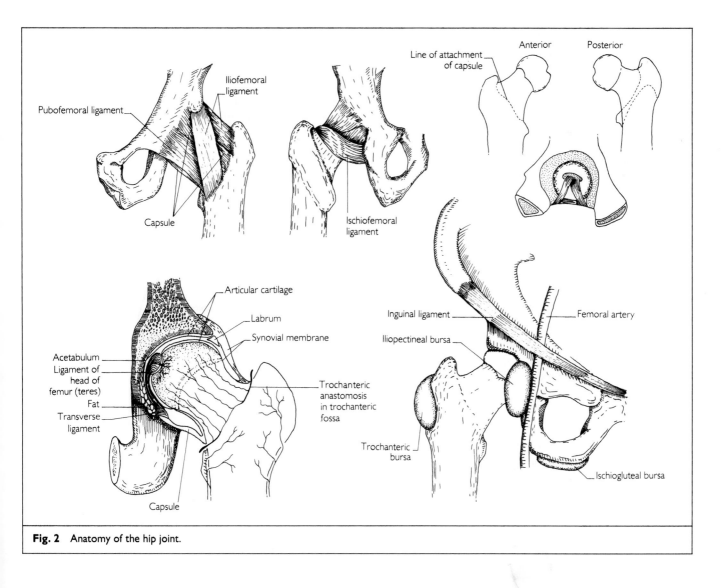

Fig. 2 Anatomy of the hip joint.

chanteric bursa and the ischiogluteal bursa. The iliopectineal bursa lies over the anterior surface of the articular capsule beneath the deep surface of the iliopsoas muscle and between the iliofemoral and pubofemoral ligaments. It is the largest and most constant of the bursae and communicates with the hip joint in approximately 15%. The trochanteric bursa is multilocular and situated between the posterolateral surface of the greater trochanter and the gluteus maximus muscle. The ischiogluteal bursa is over the ischial tuberosity and overlies the sciatic nerve.

The hip joint is surrounded by powerful muscle groups which maintain the upright position of the trunk and assist locomotion. They are summarised in Table 1.

Table I. Muscle groups of the hip joint

Movement	Muscle group	Nerve root supply
Flexion		
Prime	Iliopsoas	
Accessory	Rectus femoris	
	Pectineus	L2,3
	Sartorius	
	Adductor longus	
Extension		
Prime	Gluteus maximus	
	Hamstrings	
Accessory	Ischial head of	L4,5, S1,2
	adductor magnus	
Abduction		
Prime	Gluteus medius	
Accessory	Gluteus minimus	L4,5, S1
Adduction		
Prime	Adductor magnus	
	Adductor longus	
	Adductor brevis	L3,4,5, S1
	Pectineus	
	Gracilis	
External rotation		
Prime	Gluteus maximus	
	Quadratus femoris	
	Piriformis	L4,5, S1
Accessory	Sartorius	
	Gracilis	
Internal rotation		
Prime	Gluteus minimus	
Accessory	Gluteus medius	
	Adductor longus	
	Adductor brevis	L4,5, S1
	Adductor magnus	
	Pectineus	
	Iliacus	
	Psoas	

Symptoms

Pain is the most common complaint although some severe disorders of the hip, such as congenital dislocation and congenital coxa vara, are typically painless. Limping and other functional deficiencies can be a major feature whether or not the hip is painful. Common disabilities are difficulty getting out of bed in the morning, reaching to put on socks, climbing stairs and sexual intercourse.

The innervation of the leg is shown in Figure 3. Pain from the hip joint is often ill-defined and may be felt in the groin, inner thigh, trochanteric area, buttock, anterior thigh and knee (Fig. 4). The reason why patients may present with knee pain is that both the hip and the knee receive a nerve supply from the obturator nerve and the femoral nerve. Pain from the joint therefore needs to be differentiated from referred pain from lumbar spinal disease and meralgia paraesthetica, and from that due to sacroiliitis, trochanteric bursitis, ischial bursitis and adductor tendinitis (Fig. 4b).

In diseases of the articular surface, pain is often aggravated by weight-bearing. Pain due to joint inflammation is accompanied by prolonged stiffness and is often relieved by holding the leg in slight flexion if the joint capsule is distended. Pain resulting from joint infection or bone disease such as osteoid osteoma is often worse at night. The pain of bursitis is usually

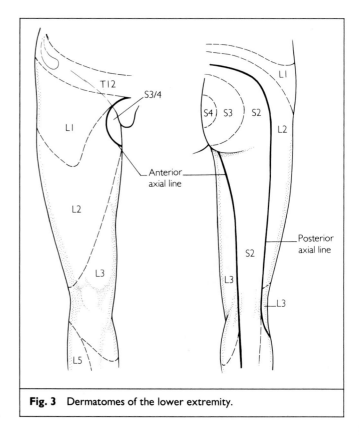

Fig. 3 Dermatomes of the lower extremity.

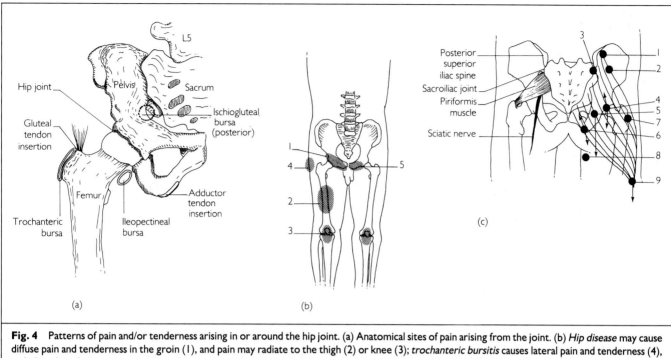

Fig. 4 Patterns of pain and/or tenderness arising in or around the hip joint. (a) Anatomical sites of pain arising from the joint. (b) *Hip disease* may cause diffuse pain and tenderness in the groin (1), and pain may radiate to the thigh (2) or knee (3); *trochanteric bursitis* causes lateral pain and tenderness (4), and *gluteal tendinitis* may cause pain in the same area on resisted abduction; *adductor tendinitis* causes pain in the groin on resisted adduction (5); *meralgia paraesthetica* causes pain and dysaesthesia in a patch on the front of the thigh (2). (c) Posterior view; note the gluteus maximus attaching to the iliotibial tract: 1, gluteus medius bursa; 2, gluteus medius and maximus trigger point; 3, sacroiliac joint; 4, hip joint; 5, sciatic nerve; 6, ischiogluteal bursa; 7 trochanteric bursa; 8, adductor tendons; 9, iliotibial tract.

more localised. Trochanteric bursitis is aggravated by lying on the affected side, whereas the pain from ischiogluteal bursitis is worse when sitting.

Examination

Inspection

The patient is undressed to underpants and examined walking, standing and lying. Easily identifiable bony landmarks of the pelvis and femur (Fig. 5) are the crest of the ilium, which terminates anteriorly at the anterior superior spine and posteriorly at the posterior superior spine, the ischial tuberosity and the greater trochanter. Anteriorly, the hip joint is beneath a point 3 cm below the midpoint of the inguinal ligament and 3 cm lateral to the palpable femoral artery.

Walking into the clinic the patient may give away the presence of hip disease. An antalgic gait indicates a painful hip. During the phase of gait when weight-bearing is on the affected side, the body leans over to

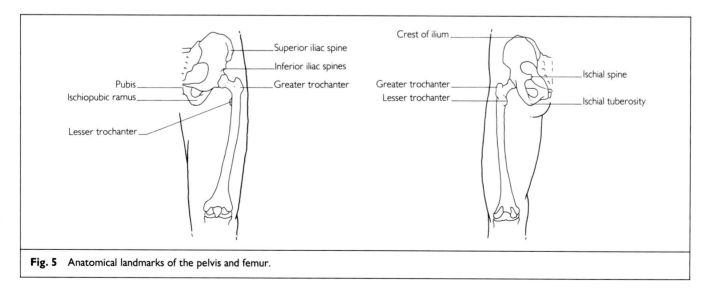

Fig. 5 Anatomical landmarks of the pelvis and femur.

the affected side to avoid painful contraction of the hip abductors. A Trendelenburg gait, on the other hand, indicates weakness of the abductor muscles, which is a frequent occurrence in any chronic hip disease. Here the pelvis on the opposite side drops and the body leans away from the affected side when weight-bearing is on the diseased hip. A waddling gait due to bilateral chronic hip disease and abductor muscle weakness is very typical of bilateral congenital hip displacement.

With the patient standing it is helpful to have him or her point to the site of pain. From the front, a pelvic tilt can be detected from the level of the anterior iliac spines (Fig. 6(a)). This is due to adduction or abduction deformity resulting from hip disease, a short leg or primary scoliosis. External rotation, which is common in severe osteoarthritis or femoral neck fracture, may be apparent. From the side (Fig. 6(b)) an exaggerated lumbar lordosis may be an indication of a fixed flexion deformity of one or both hips. From behind (Fig. 6(c)), elevation of the iliac crest and the gluteal fold on one side may indicate hip deformity. With fixed adduction, the diseased side is elevated and the patient may be unable to stand with the foot of the involved leg flat on the floor. With an abduction deformity the situation is reversed. Muscle wasting may be apparent, as the result of disuse in hip disease or due to primary neurological or muscle involvement.

The *Trendelenburg test* (Fig. 7) detects weakness of the gluteus medius hip abductors. This can be due to a variety of chronic hip diseases or to primary neurological or muscle disorders. The patient is asked to stand on the affected hip. Normally, the centre of gravity is brought over the weight-bearing foot and the abductor muscles hold the pelvis level or even with the non-supporting side slightly elevated. A positive test is indicated by dropping of the non-weight-bearing side.

When the patient is lying supine with the pelvis as level as possible, leg-length discrepancy will be obvious. Measuring each leg from the anterior iliac spine to the medial malleolus will indicate true leg shortening. A difference of less than 1 cm is quite commonly encountered and does not produce a functional problem. With a fixed adduction deformity, the affected leg may cross the normal one. Rotational deformities may be obvious, and an inflamed, painful hip tends to be held in slight flexion, abduction and external rotation.

The hip joint is deep-seated and joint swelling is not usually apparent. Occasionally, swelling of the iliopectineal bursa can be seen in the medial part of the groin.

Palpation

Use the inguinal ligament (anterior superior iliac spine to pubis) and femoral artery as landmarks. Below the middle third of the inguinal ligament and just lateral to the femoral artery pulse, the anterior part of the hip joint can be palpated where a small part of the head

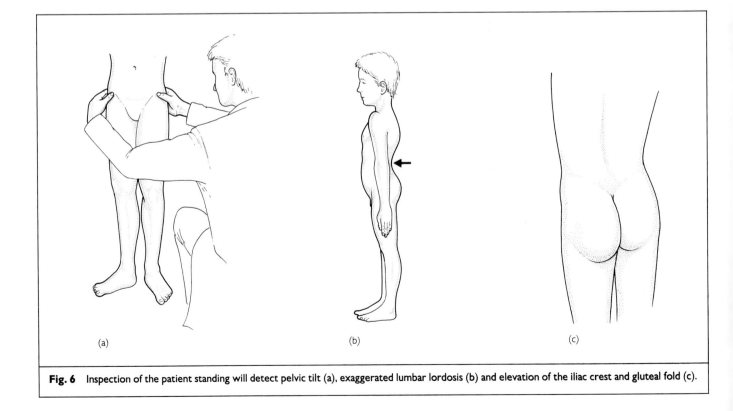

(a)   (b)   (c)

Fig. 6   Inspection of the patient standing will detect pelvic tilt (a), exaggerated lumbar lordosis (b) and elevation of the iliac crest and gluteal fold (c).

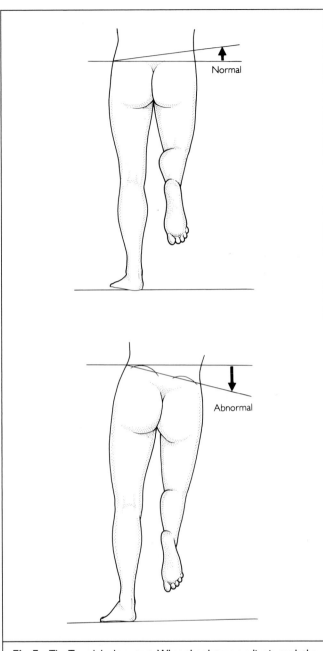

Fig. 7 The Trendelenburg test. When the gluteus medius is weak the pelvis drops on the nonweight-bearing side when the patient stands on the affected hip (lower).

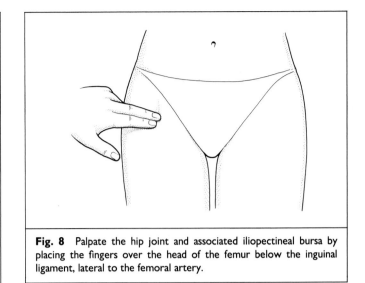

Fig. 8 Palpate the hip joint and associated iliopectineal bursa by placing the fingers over the head of the femur below the inguinal ligament, lateral to the femoral artery.

lateral cutaneous nerve of the thigh penetrates the deep fascia, is typical of meralgia paraesthetica. This is an entrapment neuropathy of this nerve.

By flexing and abducting the hip (Fig. 9), tenderness due to adductor tendinitis can be detected. Tenderness around the symphysis pubis and inferior pubic ramus occurs in spondylarthropathies as a result of enthesitis.

Turn the patient on his or her side to palpate the greater trochanter. Bursitis causes tenderness over the lateral aspect of the greater trochanter and occasionally there is swelling. Tenderness of the tendon insertions occurs on the posterolateral aspect of the greater trochanter. To palpate the ischial tuberosity, flex the hip and knee (Fig. 10). Tenderness may indicate bursitis, and rheumatoid nodules may be felt at

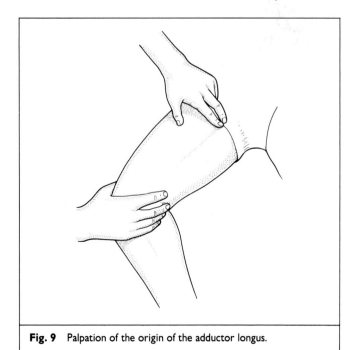

Fig. 9 Palpation of the origin of the adductor longus.

lies outside the acetabulum. Overlying this is the iliopectineal bursa. Tenderness at this site (Fig. 8) may be due to joint inflammation or bursitis. Swelling of the iliopectineal bursa may be felt. This may be due to a localized bursitis or may represent a synovial cyst through communication with an underlying inflamed hip joint. Swelling of the bursa must be distinguished from other swellings in this region, particularly from a femoral hernia that lies medial to the femoral artery.

Localised tenderness approximately 10 cm below the anterior superior iliac crest, at the point where the

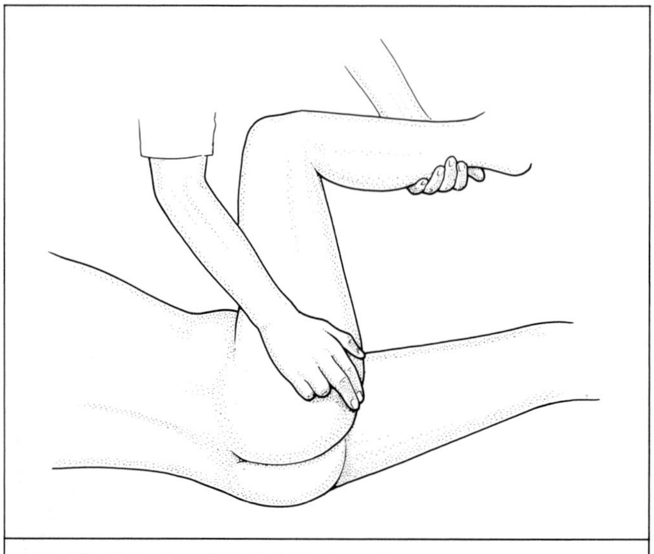

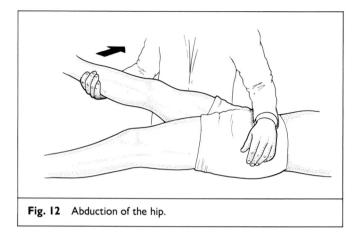

Fig. 12   Abduction of the hip.

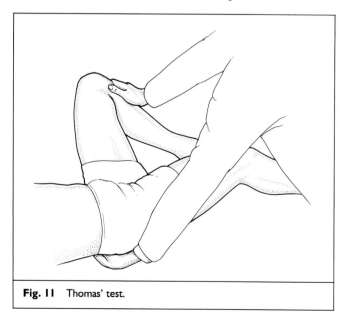

Fig. 10   Palpation of the ischial tuberosity.

this site. The sciatic nerve can be palpated midway between the greater trochanter and the ischial tuberosity and is tender in conditions putting pressure on it, such as intervertebral disc disease.

With the leg extended, percussion of the heel of the foot with the examiner's hand can produce pain in the hip in early cases of hip disease (the 'anvil' test).

Range of movements

Except for testing extension, movements of the hip are best determined with the patient lying supine. The normal range of movements varies from person to person.

Thomas' test indicates a fixed flexion deformity of the hip (Fig. 11). Flex the good hip fully, observing with the other hand that the lumbar spine is flattened.

Fig. 11   Thomas' test.

Lifting of the thigh on the affected side with flexion of the knee indicates a positive test.

The range of flexion (approximately 120°) is tested with the knees flexed. Flexion of the hip with the knee extended is limited by tension in the hamstrings and varies considerably from person to person, from over 90° to less than 75°.

Abduction is frequently lost in hip disease. Test this with the legs extended by stabilising the pelvis with a hand on the opposite anterior iliac crest (Fig. 12) and grasping the ankle with the other hand. The hip is abducted until the pelvis tilts (approximately 45°). Additionally, the examiner can stand at the end of the couch to grasp both ankles and simultaneously abduct both hips: one can better appreciate differences between the two hips and measure the intermalleolar distance for future comparison. Adduction is assessed by crossing one leg over the other; normally, approximately 30° is possible before the pelvis tilts.

Loss of internal rotation is one of the earliest and most reliable signs of hip disease. Test this by flexing the hip and knee to 90° and rotate the foot laterally (Fig. 13). Normally there is about 45° of internal rotation but this is reduced with ageing, therefore a difference between the two sides is important. External rotation (approximately 45°, Fig. 14) is tested by rotating the foot medially. A rough idea of internal and external rotation and a comparison between the two sides can be achieved with the legs extended (Fig. 15), rolling each leg first one way then the other.

Extension of the hip is checked with the patient lying prone. The examiner partially immobilises the pelvis and lumbar spine by applying downward pressure with one hand while extending the hip with the other hand placed on the anterior aspect of the thigh.

Pain on resisted movements in association with localised pain and tenderness indicates a tendinitis. For example, pain on resisted adduction and resisted abduction is typical of adductor tendinitis and gluteal tendinitis respectively.

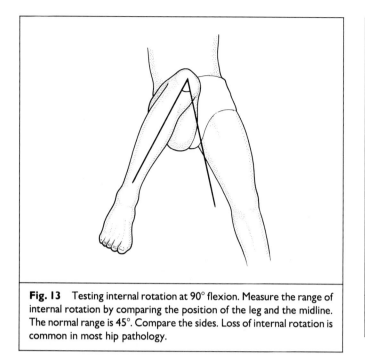

Fig. 13 Testing internal rotation at 90° flexion. Measure the range of internal rotation by comparing the position of the leg and the midline. The normal range is 45°. Compare the sides. Loss of internal rotation is common in most hip pathology.

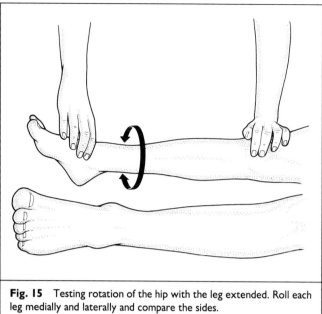

Fig. 15 Testing rotation of the hip with the leg extended. Roll each leg medially and laterally and compare the sides.

Muscle testing

Flexors of the hip are best tested with the patient sitting with his or her legs hanging over the couch. The hip is then actively flexed against graded resistance. The internal and external rotators are then tested with one of the examiner's hands applying counter-pressure to the thigh and the other hand applying graded resistance above the ankle against the movement being tested (Fig. 16).

Abductors and adductors are tested with the patient

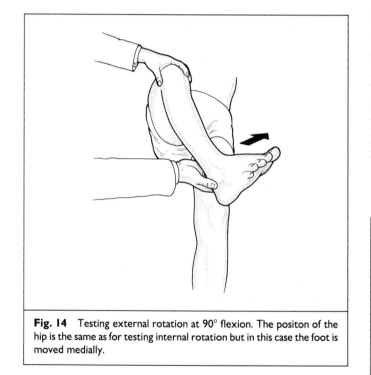

Fig. 14 Testing external rotation at 90° flexion. The positon of the hip is the same as for testing internal rotation but in this case the foot is moved medially.

The *Ober test* demonstrates contraction of the iliotibial band. The patient lies on his or her side and the underneath hip is flexed to eliminate lordosis of the lumbar spine. The knee of the upper leg is flexed to 90°, and the thigh is abducted and extended. In a positive test, when the examiner's supporting hand is removed, the hip remains abducted rather than dropping back to the couch and the iliotibial band is often palpated as a rigid band in the subcutaneous tissues below the iliac crest.

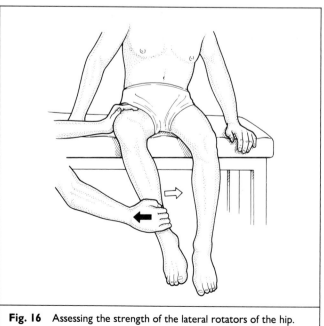

Fig. 16 Assessing the strength of the lateral rotators of the hip.

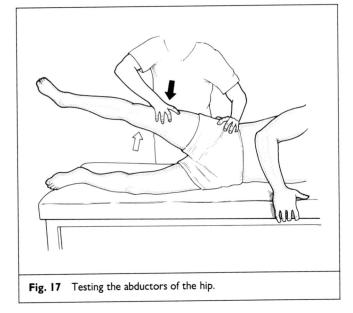

Fig. 17 Testing the abductors of the hip.

on one side with legs extended. For the abductors (Fig. 17), the lower leg is slightly flexed to maintain balance, the pelvis is stablised with one hand, the upper leg is extended slightly and the patient abducts the leg against resistance provided by the examiner's other hand.

To test the adductors (Fig. 18), the upper leg is supported in approximately 30° of abduction, and adduction of the lower leg is resisted by the examiner with the other hand above the knee.

Testing the extensors is performed with the patient prone and the legs extended. With one hand on the sacrum to hold the pelvis down, the examiner resists extension of the hip with the other hand above the knee.

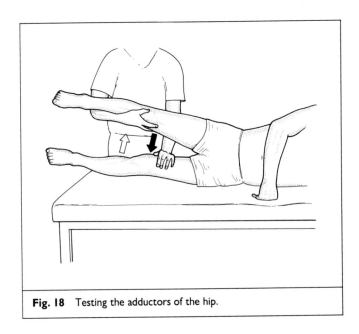

Fig. 18 Testing the adductors of the hip.

Local Aspiration and Injection

Hip joint

Aspiration of the hip joint requires more skill than other sites because the joint is deep to the skin surface so that one is unable to feel the articulation between the bones and often unable to confirm that the needle is in the joint space. The procedure is easier if fluoroscopy is available.

Figure 19 shows the anterior approach. The needle is inserted two fingers width lateral to the femoral artery, just below the inguinal ligament.

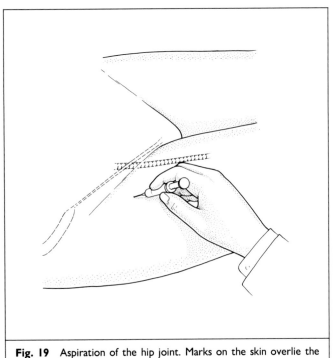

Fig. 19 Aspiration of the hip joint. Marks on the skin overlie the anterior superior spine, the greater trochanter, the femoral artery, and the inguinal ligament. The needle is inserted two fingers width lateral to the femoral artery, just below the inguinal ligament.

Bursitis

Trochanteric bursitis
With the affected side uppermost, identify the tender site over the trochanteric prominence. The needle is inserted perpendicular to the skin until the trochanter is reached and then withdrawn slightly.

Ischiogluteal bursitis
Locate the site of greatest tenderness, with the patient on his or her side, and inject into this.

Meralgia paraesthetica (Fig. 20)

Locate the tender spot where the lateral cutaneous nerve of the thigh penetrates the fascia of the upper thigh approximately 10 cm below the anterior superior iliac crest. This site is then infiltrated.

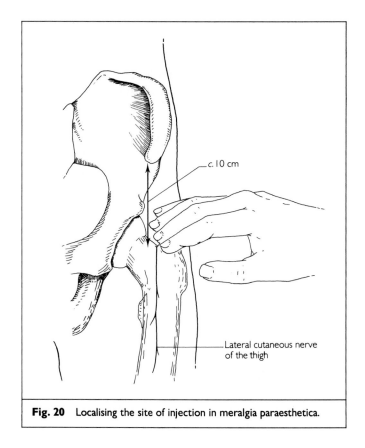

c. 10 cm

Lateral cutaneous nerve of the thigh

Fig. 20 Localising the site of injection in meralgia paraesthetica.

6

THE KNEE

The knee is the largest and most complicated joint in the body and is a modified hinge joint with two tibiofemoral components and one patellofemoral. In some lower mammals, three distinct synovial cavities are found.

The knee is not constrained by the shape of its bones; it depends for stability on internal (cruciates and menisci) and external soft tissues (capsule and capsular ligaments) and muscle function/co-ordination. Nevertheless, the knee remains relatively unstable and is the joint most susceptible to injury, osteochondritis dissecans, loose bodies and synovial chondromatosis. The peripheral joint involvement of the seronegative spondarthritides typically includes the knee and symmetrical knee joint synovitis in rheumatoid arthritis is common.

It is the easiest joint to aspirate and therefore a frequent site for diagnostic aspiration.

Development

Prenatal development

The development of the knee has been studied more than that of any other joint. By approximately 8 weeks it resembles that of the adult in form, the patella being cartilaginous by 10 weeks. The cruciate ligaments and menisci develop *in situ* and are not therefore secondary capsular structures. The characteristic feature of synovial tissue in the fetus is a vascularised loose connective tissue, covered by synovial cells of varied arrangements. A fibrous capsule is present only in the posterior part of the joint, and its appearance is so variable that it does not appear a necessary prelude to the formation of intra-articular structures.

Developmental abnormalities

The knee is commonly the site of abnormality in the disorders of epiphyseal growth. Where such a disorder is suspected it is essential to assess the whole skeletal system, to compare the findings with normal clinical and radiological charts and then refer to one of the specialist texts (e.g. *Atlas of Skeletal Dysplasias*). *Genu varum* or *valgum* may be found according to the

main site of epiphyseal maldevelopment. Where major laxity is a feature, recurvatum is likely.

Minor genu varum is common in normal children before the age of 3 years, and genu valgum may continue until 7 years. Severe genu valgum is seen in *Morquio's* syndrome due to failure of ossification of the lateral side of the upper tibial epiphyses. *Hypochondroplasia* (prevalence 3–4 per million), when severe, is indistinguishable from *achondroplasia*, but the only lower limb finding in the mild form may be genu varum (8% of cases).

Pseudoachondroplasia (prevalence 4 per million), unlike achondroplasia, causes marked epiphyseal and metaphyseal involvement, leading to premature osteoarthritis.

In *Marfan's syndrome* there is joint laxity and knee recurvatum, in addition to the long bone excess.

Functional Anatomy

The knee is a modified hinge joint that also shows gliding and rotation of the articular surfaces on each other. The femoral condyles are *convex*, accentuated posteriorly. The tibial condyles are hollowed centrally but flattened peripherally so that concavity is produced by the overlying semilunar cartilages (*menisci*). Stability is therefore provided by the internal (*cruciate ligaments* and *menisci*) and external (*capsule* and *capsular ligaments*) soft tissues, including coordinated muscle function.

Menisci

The menisci (Fig. 1) or semilunar cartilages, are crescent-shaped portions of fibrocartilage, producing concavity by their situation on the upper articular surface of the tibia. Since they are wedge-shaped in cross-section, they match the adjacent articular surfaces of the femur and tibia.

Meniscal function

The menisci have a mild stabilising effect, exert some restriction on excessive lateral movement and facilitate the 'screw-home' movement. They act as 'thrust pads' aiding lubrication. They also play an important role in

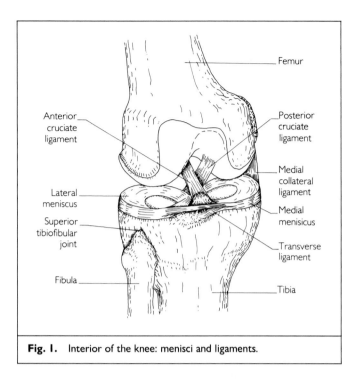

Fig. I.   Interior of the knee: menisci and ligaments.

load-bearing, transmitting up to 70% of weight in extension through the lateral side and 50% medially.

Fibrous capsule

There is no defined complete capsule, but rather a thick ligamentous sheath comprising mainly tendons or expansions from them.

Anterior

- Fused tendons of the rectus femoris and vasti insert into the upper patella, with superficial fibres continuing over the anterior patella into the ligamentum patellae.
- Thinner bands from the sides of the patella attach to the anterior border of each tibial condyle (*medial and lateral patellar retinacula*).
- Strong expansions of fascia lata lie more superficially (*iliotibial tract*), descending over the anterolateral knee to the lateral tibial condyle, with a band to the lateral upper patella (*superior patellar retinaculum*).

Note: Unlike other hinge joints the 'capsule' is continuous with the muscle above, so its tension can be fully modified in all positions.

Posterior

- True capsular fibres attach to the femur above the condyles and to the intercondylar line, vertically down to the upper tibia.
- Centrally strengthened by the *oblique popliteal ligament.*
- Inferolaterally by the *arcuate popliteal ligament.*

Medial

- The true capsular fibres form the *superficial collateral ligament*, which is broad and flat attaching to the medial epicondyle of the femur, passing down and slightly forwards to the medial tibia (superficial to below tibial tubercle, deep also to medial meniscus).
- Expansions of *semimembranosus tendon* add considerable strength to the medial and posterior capsule.

Lateral

- The *fibular collateral ligament* is round and cord-like, separated from the lateral capsule and enclosed by an expansion of fascia lata. It splits the tendon of biceps femoris.
- The popliteus tendon lies between the lateral meniscus and capsule.

Note: the collateral ligaments are most tightly stretched in extension, and their lines of attachment prevent rotation of the tibia laterally or of the femur medially in extension. Rotation is easily demonstrated in the flexed knee.

Intra-articular ligaments

These are called *cruciates* as they cross each other within the joint.

Anterior cruciate (ACL)

This extends obliquely up and back from the anterior intercondylar area of the tibia to the medial aspect of lateral femoral condyle. Thus it prevents posterior displacement of the femur on the tibia.

Posterior cruciate (PCL)

This is less oblique, shorter and stronger. It passes up and forwards from the posterior intercondylar area of the tibia medial to the ACL, and attaches to the lateral side of medial femoral condyle. It prevents anterior displacement of the femur on the tibia.

These ligaments are more taut in extension and tend to rotate the tibia laterally. They tighten when the tibia is rotated medially and slacken when rotated laterally as the ligaments uncross.

Extensor mechanism (Fig.2)

Extension is by the quadriceps femoris, which is one of the most powerful muscles in the body. It is formed by the rectus femoris and three vasti (medialis, intermedius and lateralis), and extends the knee and flexes the hip.

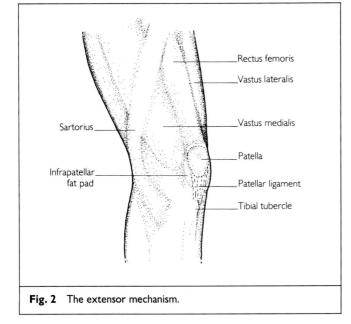

Fig. 2   The extensor mechanism.

Any injury to the knee joint produces inhibition of this muscle, which rapidly loses bulk, tone and control, especially seen in the vastus medialis obliquus (VMO). The VMO is the most important component and contributes to medial stability of patella and the 'screw home' movement of the femur on the tibia in the last 10° of extension.

The *patellar ligament* is an extension of the quadriceps (patellar) tendon from the inferior patellar pole to its insertion into the tibial tubercle. The infrapatellar fat pad can be seen on either side of the ligament, as it lies behind the ligament, separating it from the synovial membrane.

Knee flexion is performed by the hamstrings (biceps femoris, semimembranosus and semitendinosus) and gastrocnemii.

- *The biceps femoris* by its insertion to fibular head, fibular collateral ligament, iliotibial tract and upper tibia and deep fascia of the calf, flexes the knee and gives lateral dynamic support.
- *The semimembranosus*, by its insertion to posterior and medial tibial condyle and post capsule, flexes and gives posterior and medial stability. Its tendon extends across the posterior aspect from the medial tibial condyle upwards to the lateral femoral condyle as the *posterior oblique ligament*.
- *The semitendinosus* joins the sartorius to insert into upper and medial tibial shaft and *gracilis* (pes anserinus).

Rotation

Rotation is not possible in the fully extended stable knee; but as the knee flexes, medial rotation is per-

formed by the sartorius, gracilis, semimembranosus and semitendinosus. Lateral rotation is carried out by the biceps femoris and tensor fasciae latae.

Rotatory stability

Rotatory stability is provided by the popliteus, which is a medial rotator of the tibia on the femur and protects the posterolateral portion of the lateral meniscus, because the tendon attaches to the lateral meniscus and pulls it back during knee flexion and medial rotation.

Medial stability

Medial stability (Fig. 3) is achieved by the function of the medial collateral ligament, which is a primary static stabiliser, and the semimembranosus muscle, which is a dynamic stabiliser. The medial tibial collateral ligament is phylogenetically a continuation of the insertion of the adductor magnus. It comprises a superficial portion, a deep portion (from the joint capsule and attaching to the peripheral medial meniscus), and an oblique portion which is fan-shaped from the medial femoral condyle to the posterior tract of the medial tibial condyle and peripheral medial meniscus. The oblique portion remains tight in flexion, when the posterior capsule is very lax.

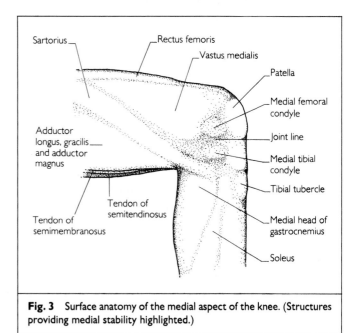

Fig. 3   Surface anatomy of the medial aspect of the knee. (Structures providing medial stability highlighted.)

Lateral stability

Lateral stability (Fig. 4) is achieved by the function of the lateral (fibular) collateral ligament as a static stabiliser and the biceps femoris muscle as a dynamic

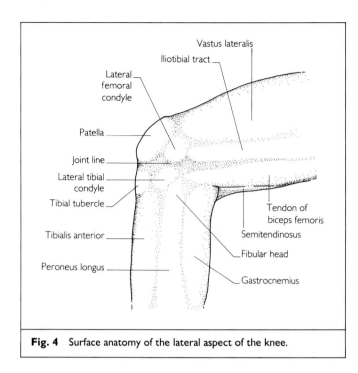

Fig. 4 Surface anatomy of the lateral aspect of the knee.

stabiliser. The lateral collateral ligament is phylogenetically the origin of the peroneus longus, and it extends from the lateral epicondyle of the femur down to the head of the fibula. It splits the tendon of the biceps femoris and is separated from the lateral meniscus by the tendon of popliteus.

Innervation

The knee joint is supplied by several branches of the femoral nerve, the common peroneal and tibial (sciatic) nerves and a filament from the obturator nerve. The latter explains the common referral to the pain of hip joint disease as knee pain, typically medially.

Vascular supply

There are branches from the popliteal, anterior tibial and a descending branch from the lateral circumflex femoral branch of the arteria profunda femoris.

Pain Patterns in the Knee

It is necessary to define whether symptoms are spontaneous or post-traumatic. The features of inflammatory or degenerative joint disease have been outlined in Chapter 1.

Osteoarthritis

Pain is usually first noticed on exercise, but can initially be 'walked off'. The patient may complain that the knee creaks and grates, with episodes of swelling, particularly after unusual activity in a flexed position (e.g. squatting or kneeling). The swelling and a variable degree of inflammatory response in the synovium produces a stiff, tight feeling (*inactivity stiffness*), felt particularly at the back of the knee. Sudden increase in stress may precipitate acute pain. Cartilage or osteophytic fragments which separate into the joint may cause loose body *locking*. Flexion deformity occurs due to protective hamstring spasm but will in time become a fixed flexion deformity.

In the later stages, pain becomes more severe and near constant, with progressive genu varum. The patient becomes unable to squat or kneel and has difficulty climbing stairs.

Synovitis

The patient complains of pain and stiffness with marked morning symptoms. Tightness at the back of the knee may be very limiting, particularly if there is a tense popliteal cyst. If the effusion is very tense, flexion is often very restricted and extension difficult due to hamstring tightness. Flexion contracture will develop if the effects are not reduced by reduction of synovitis and splintage.

History of Injury

It is important to define the history of the plane and forces of injury.

Acute injury

A team doctor, coach or physiotherapist may be able to describe the observed forces of injury. It is vital to examine the injured knee immediately before protective muscle spasm makes this impossible. *Immediate swelling* indicates a haemarthrosis and demands urgent investigation to determine whether it is due to cruciate ligament tear, osteochondral injury or other pathology.

Chronic injury

The history of the type of injury may be the main pointer to the likely damage, as physical signs are often of limited value. The patient should be asked to describe or demonstrate the pattern of injury. Where no defined injury is recalled, the loading, type of training and surfaces used should be defined.

An alternative pathology must be considered if the symptoms and signs do not fit with the stresses involved.

Anterior knee pain

Pain is felt behind the knee cap, particularly after sitting with the knee flexed for some time (cinema sign), and is relieved by movement but aggravated by heavy exercise especially loaded in flexion. There is pain particularly when descending stairs. This is because of increased stress on this compartment, when maintaining knee flexion or particularly when weight-bearing on a flexed knee.

In the examination:

- the findings are often minimal,
- there is tenderness of the medial patella undersurface,
- fluid and crepitus may be present in chondromalacia patellae if severe.

'Giving way' due to patellar subluxation

The patella functions in a state of dynamic equilibrium between lateral forces (vastus lateralis, bony contour and position of tibial tubercle and genu valgum) and medial forces (patella alta, ligamentous laxity and vastus medialis).

In *mild* patellar subluxation, the patella slips momentarily over the condyle. The patient describes the history of 'giving way' and may develop mild synovitis or effusion after each episode, if infrequent. Frequent displacement is, on the other hand, often pain-free.

The patellar apprehension test: The examiner pushes the patella laterally with the knee in extension; as the knee is flexed actively, the patient resists further flexion because of fear of painful dislocation. A positive test is strong evidence of recurrent dislocation, in patients presenting with a history of recurrent 'giving way' of the knee. However, apprehension may also be seen in individuals complaining of patellofemoral pain without a history of 'giving way'.

In *major* subluxation with severe pain, reduction under general anaesthesia is usually necessary when the episode is the first and due to direct injury. Arthroscopy should be performed to exclude injury to the patella surface, since later symptoms due to a detached osteochondral fragment may develop.

Vastus medialis obliquus wasting is often a prominent finding in patients with patellar abnormalities.

Medial meniscal tear

Acute: there is usually a history of an outward twist of foot/ankle or an inward twist of femur on fixed foot with the knee in flexion. Immediate anteromedial pain is often sufficient to make the individual collapse. There may have been a feeling of a tearing sensation inside the joint. On attempting to stand, the knee usually cannot be straightened *if* there is displacement of the meniscal segment. Swelling develops a few hours later (*unless* there is cruciate tear, when immediate swelling, due to haemarthrosis, occurs), and over 1 week the symptoms tend to improve, but chronic symptoms may be noted.

Chronic: the patient can usually walk and carry out normal activities, but any twisting movement gives pain or *giving way of the knee*. Locking episodes and recurrent small effusions may also be noticed, but persistent effusion is relatively uncommon. Quadriceps wasting is common.

Lateral meniscal tear

The history is usually similar except that the pain is often felt posteriorly, locking is less frequent and the injury sometimes remains asymptomatic.

Locked knee

Locking refers to the inability to fully extend the knee (*blocked knee*) due to a meniscal tear, or to hyperextend it if it normally does. *Fixed flexion deformity* is the clinical sign, and the affected knee should be compared with the normal one. *Locking* due to a *loose body*, occurs suddenly in mid-movement and prevents extension or flexion. Sudden intense pain may cause the patient to fall. Typically the site of pain is variable. Recurrent episodes may lead to chronic synovitis and effusion.

Examination

As with all lower limb joints, assessment should begin with observation of standing posture, gait and leg length. Observe the alignment between the lower leg (tibia) and upper leg (femur).

Genu varum

Genu varum (*see* Chapter 1) refers to lateral curvature of the leg involving tibia or tibia and femur:

- *Tibia: physiological tibial bowing* refers to minor bowing, which is common before the age of 3 years; it corrects with further growth. *Pathological tibial bowing* results from rickets, typically in the distal third, trauma or infection.
- *Tibia/femur:* congenital genu varum occurs because of abnormalities in epiphyseal growth. In osteoarthritis genu varum develops when there is loss of the medial compartment cartilage and ligament laxity.

Genu valgum (*See* Chapter 1)

- *Physiological* genu valgum resolves by the age of 7 years.
- *Unilateral* genu valgum may be due to trauma, infections, congenital causes affecting epiphyseal growth.
- *Bilateral (or unilateral)* genu valgum is usually a result of inflammatory joint disease, for example rheumatoid arthritis.

Genu recurvatum

This is hyperextension of the knee beyond 10° (Fig. 5) and may be part of a generalised hypermobility syndrome or localised causes, including under-development of the femoral condyles or relaxation of the posterior capsular structures and weakness in the calf and hamstring muscles.

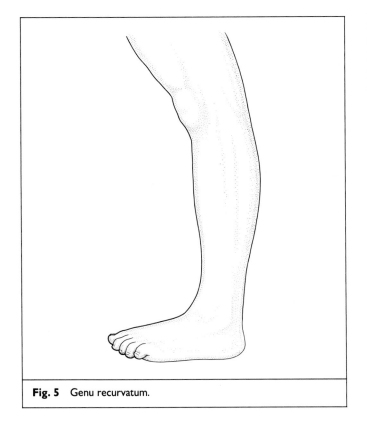

Fig. 5 Genu recurvatum.

Muscle wasting

Observe the quadriceps muscle bulk, the vastus medialis particularly as it wastes rapidly in any painful knee condition. Exclude evidence of denervation, root irritation (positive femoral stretch test) or primary muscle disease (myopathy/myositis). Compare muscle strength in quadriceps with hamstrings, as

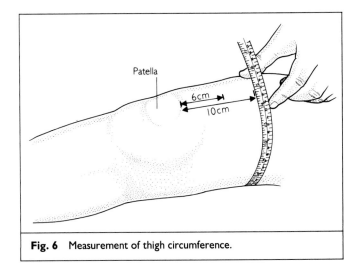

Fig. 6 Measurement of thigh circumference.

imbalance may be the cause of persistent problems, particularly in sportsmen.

A tape-measure record of muscle wasting can be made by a circumferential measure at a point (6–10 cm) measured and marked above the superior patellar pole on both sides (Fig. 6). Reproducibility is rather poor, but serial measurements may have some value in monitoring recovery of muscle bulk. *Maximum* calf circumference is more reproducible.

Swelling

Define whether there is *generalised* (e.g. effusion or soft tissue) or *localised* (e.g. meniscal or bursal) swelling.

Effusion

This fills in the parapatellar gutters and suprapatellar pouch, but also examine for popliteal swelling. A small effusion is best defined by the *bulge test*. Fluid is stroked by the palm of the (right) hand from the medial joint-line (start at tibial condyle) upwards into the suprapatellar pouch (Fig. 7). The (left) hand is immediately placed across the upper medial line with the thumb resting on the patella, thus controlling the fluid in the pouch. The fluid is then stroked down from the suprapatellar pouch by the dorsum of the right hand running down the lateral joint-line.

A bulge of fluid at the medial patellar gutter confirms a small effusion (Fig. 7(d)). This must be defined from movement of the patella or soft tissues, but this should be controlled by the thumb resting on the patella.

A large effusion can be defined by cross-fluctuance or the patellar tap test, provided the effusion has not become very tense.

The patellar tap (Fig. 8): the left hand controls the effusion by pressure over the suprapatellar pouch,

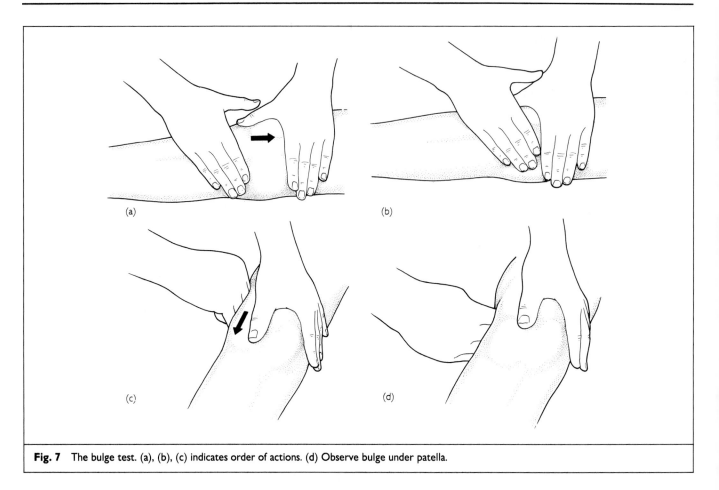

Fig. 7 The bulge test. (a), (b), (c) indicates order of actions. (d) Observe bulge under patella.

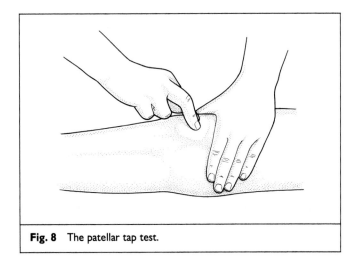

Fig. 8 The patellar tap test.

Localised swelling

The examiner should define

- anatomical site,
- communication with the knee joint,
- reducibility,
- consistency,
- tenderness,
- transillumination,
- and also exclude pulsatilion (also examine for bruit).

Bursae

The bursae of the knee are illustrated in Figure 9.

while the right hand (index and middle fingers) taps the patella against the underlying femur by a sharp downward pressure with the knee in extension.

Synovitis can be crudely assessed by palpating the thickness of tissue in the suprapatellar pouch below the main quadriceps bulk, or by palpating swelling at the anterior joint line which immediately reforms after pressure although this may be simulated by fat.

Prepatellar: this is present in about 90% of people and is subcutaneous, covering the lower half of the patella and upper half of the patellar ligament. In *bursitis due to pressure/friction* effects (housemaid's or carpet-layer's knee), pain may be absent, tenderness mild and the swelling cool. In chronic lesions the bursa may be rather indurated and gritty. In *acute bursitis*, due to crystal synovitis or sepsis, warmth, erythema and local tenderness are marked: full passive knee flexion

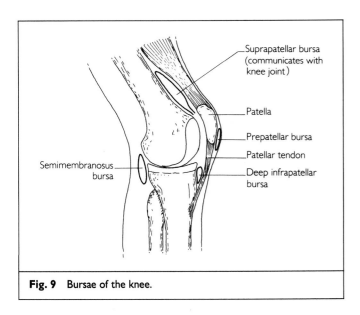

Fig. 9 Bursae of the knee.

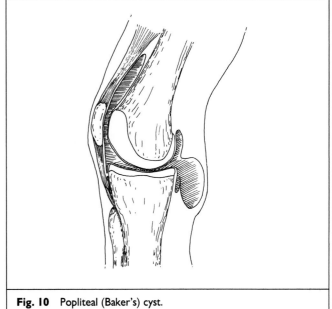

Fig. 10 Popliteal (Baker's) cyst.

may however still be possible, with discomfort at end-range, as the knee joint is not involved, being protected by dense ligamentous and fibrous structures. This is in contrast with the marked irritability and gross restriction of knee joint sepsis.

Deep infrapatellar: this small bursa lies between the upper part of the tibial tuberosity and the ligamentum patellae: it is separated from the knee joint synovium by a pad of fat. When it is inflamed, note the swelling on either side of the patellar ligament insertion to the tibial tubercle. There is pain and tenderness over the ligament, and full knee extension and flexion are not quite achieved.

Popliteus: this arises from the synovial membrane of the knee surrounding the popliteus tendon intra-articularly. When inflamed, it can be seen as a rounded swelling behind the lateral condyle of the femur, deep to biceps and the iliotibial band.

Bicipital: this is lower than the popliteus bursa, lying between the biceps tendon and the lateral ligament. It can be confused with a cyst of the lateral popliteal nerve.

Anserine: this is under the pes anserinus and therefore liable to bursitis in breast-stroke swimmers.

Semimembranosus: this lies between the head of gastrocnemius and semimembranosus, and becomes inflamed after excessive knee flexion (gamekeeper's knee). During extension the swelling is firm and tense, but in flexion it becomes soft. When it communicates with the posterior aspect of the knee joint it is usually termed a Baker's cyst (Fig. 10), which is common with a large knee joint effusion as it develops at the weak point of the posterior knee joint.

Rupture of a popliteal cyst presents with a typical history of sudden upper calf pain (the patient may describe the onset 'as if being kicked in the calf', and reduction of knee swelling, followed by generalised calf swelling and often pitting oedema of the dorsum of the foot. The most important differential diagnosis is from deep vein thrombosis, and sometimes, due to secondary venous obstruction, a deep vein thrombosis can develop after cyst rupture. A venogram is therefore the investigation of choice.

Local tenderness

Define the site—bony, soft-tissue attachment to bone (enthesis) of tendon or ligament, bursal (Fig. 9) or joint-line. Define associated swelling, and pain on resisted muscle action. Prominence and tenderness at the tibial tubercle is seen particularly in apoplysitis (Osgood–Schlatter's disease).

Patellar mechanism

Patellar position
The position of the patella is assessed by measurement of the Q-angle (Fig. 11), between the line drawn from the anterior superior iliac spine to the centre of the patella and the line of the patellar ligament to the tibial tubercle. The ratio of the patellar ligament length to patellar length should be *less than 1.2:1.0*.

The articular surface of the patella is divided into a large lateral section and smaller medial portion by a rounded vertical ridge. The cartilage cover of the most medial part of this area rests on the medial femoral condyle crescentic facet.

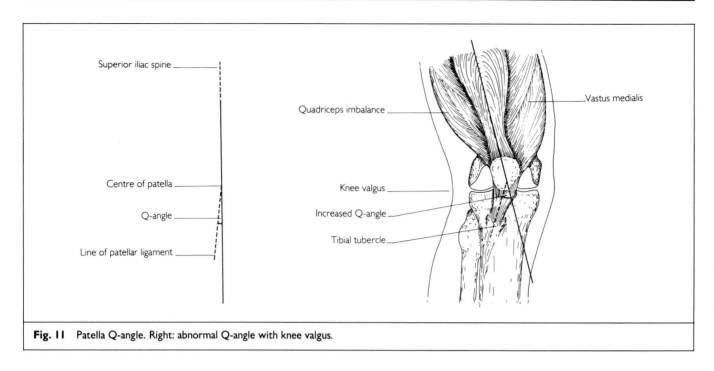

Superior iliac spine

Centre of patella

Q-angle

Line of patellar ligament

Quadriceps imbalance

Vastus medialis

Knee valgus

Increased Q-angle

Tibial tubercle

Fig. 11   Patella Q-angle. Right: abnormal Q-angle with knee valgus.

The patella tends to be displaced laterally during forced extension of the knee. This is counteracted by the buttress of the prominent lateral surface of the femur and by the retaining action of the lower fibres of vastus medialis which insert into the medial patellar border.

Abnormalities of patellar anatomy
Note any abnormalities, which include

- patella alta (high patella),
- patella baja (low patella),
- bipartite patella—a small gap may be palpable and this is usually bilateral),
- offset patella—due to an increased Q-angle.

A high patella and/or hypermobility predispose to patellar subluxation, which may follow a blow or commonly as the result of muscular action alone.

A patellar plica may be palpable, especially medially, and may be a cause of knee pain in athletes.

Range of movement and flexion deformity
Observe the position in which the knee is held. Flexion deformity or locked knee may be best detected by the prone-lying test (Fig. 12).

Quadriceps lag
Ask the patient to lift the lower limb off the couch with the knee extended. This will reveal any quadriceps lag, due to weakness. Then passively extend the knee and compare with the opposite knee. Define flexion deformity, and note that loss of hyperextension com-

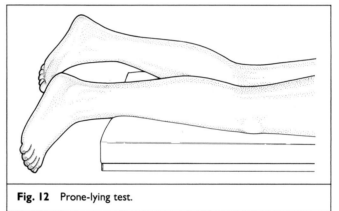

Fig. 12   Prone-lying test.

pared with the opposite side still implies a locked knee unless there is a cause for the unilateral excessive hyperextension. Then ask the patient to bend the knee as far as possible.

Flexion deformity
Define whether there is a bony or soft block to extension. The latter is a common sequel to chronic unopposed hamstring overaction with extensor weakness. Chronic hamstring tightness, particularly in sportsmen, may therefore produce flexion deformity with anterior knee pain. However, *spinal problems*, may be the underlying reason for the hamstring tightness.

Always *exclude hip flexion deformity*, which results in secondary knee flexion deformity.

Locked knee
This is usually detected easily as already outlined or by using the prone-lying test (Fig. 12). It may be due to a

meniscal tear. The site of pain on reaching the block to extension may localise the site of the tear. In a posterior horn tear of the lateral meniscus, there may be limited flexion and an audible or palpable 'clunk' on flexion. Macmurray's test for meniscal injury (rotational stress while extending the knee from almost full flexion) is not recommended as it may be very painful (including patellofemoral stress) and risks locking the meniscal fragment.

A locked knee represents a surgical emergency, because of the risk of further damage including anterior cruciate rupture. Urgent arthroscopy is indicated.

Examination for stability

Test the integrity of the collateral ligaments with the knee flexed to about 20°. The examiner controls the patient's foot and ankle between the arms and chest wall and then applies a valgus or varus stress on the tibia. Separation of the tibia from the femur at the joint-line should be checked for.

Medial collateral ligament
Valgus stretch is applied with the knee in flexion (Fig. 13) (if positive with the knee in extension, it denotes a posterior cruciate tear). Minor symmetrical stretch is normal, with up to 5 mm separation. In medial ligament injury or lesions, the following patterns are found.

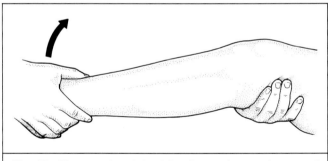

Fig. 13 The test of medial stability (arrow denotes direction of lateral stress).

- *Mild (1st degree):* there is a minimal tear with local tenderness and less than 5 mm separation (stable).
- *Moderate (2nd degree):* there is a moderate tear with marked local tenderness and between 5 and 10 mm separation.
- *Severe (3rd degree):* there is more than 10 mm separation (unstable joint).

Lateral collateral ligament
Varus stretch is applied with knee in flexion (as medial). Injury to the lateral collateral ligament is much less common than injury to the medial as adduction stress in flexion is much less frequent in sport. If it occurs, the former is usually a complex injury, with lateral capsular ligament, biceps tendon, popliteus and occasionally iliotibial tract injury.

Anterior stability
Anterior cruciate tear is best defined by the Lachman's and pivot shift tests.

Lachman's test for anterior cruciate laxity (Fig. 14): with the knee flexed to 20–30°, the femur is grasped with the left hand and the tibia with the right. Then an attempt to pull the tibia forwards (on the femur) is made.

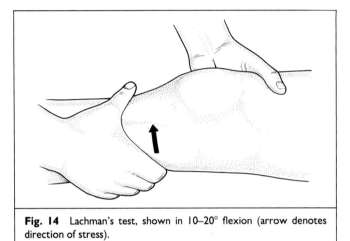

Fig. 14 Lachman's test, shown in 10–20° flexion (arrow denotes direction of stress).

Pivot shift test (Fig. 15): the lower leg, with the foot internally rotated, is supported by the examiner while applying a valgus force, as the knee is flexed from *full* extension. A tear of the anterior cruciate, because it produces anterior subluxation of the tibia on the femur, causes a jump at about 30° when the tibia reduces as the knee is flexed, sliding backwards into its correct position on the femur.

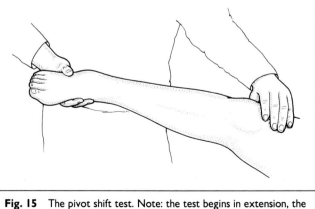

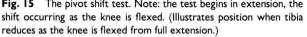

Fig. 15 The pivot shift test. Note: the test begins in extension, the shift occurring as the knee is flexed. (Illustrates position when tibia reduces as the knee is flexed from full extension.)

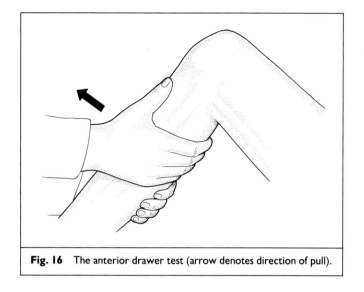

Fig. 16   The anterior drawer test (arrow denotes direction of pull).

Anterior drawer test (Fig. 16): the anterior drawer test is a less satisfactory test for anterior cruciate laxity but may have to be used by those finding the Lachman's test difficult to perform. With the knee in 90° of flexion, the examiner pulls forward with both hands on the upper posterior calf. Interpretation of the test is dependent on the position of the femur. In the neutral position it tests the capsule and anterior cruciate. With the tibia in internal rotation it tests the posterior cruciate (Fig. 16). A pure anterior drawer movement in neutral with the knee at 90° and relaxed hamstrings is termed the *anterior drawer sign*. When the tibia is internally rotated, the posterior cruciate is tight, so the anterior drawer movement cannot be achieved. Therefore a positive anterior drawer in internal rotation points to a torn posterior cruciate ligament. The interpretation of the anterior drawer test is therefore positive:

- in internal rotation—torn posterior cruciate;
- in neutral with equal tibial condyle movement—torn anterior cruciate with anteromedial/anterolateral laxity;
- in neutral with lateral tibial condyle movement—anterolateral (accentuated by the anterior cruciate);
- in neutral with medial movement: anteromedial (accentuated by anterior cruciate).

Posterior stability

The posterior drawer test is used when posterior cruciate tear is suspected. With the knee in 90° flexion, the alignment of the knee in relation to the femur is observed and compared with the opposite knee to see if there is posterior subluxation of the tibia. If there is subluxation, performing an anterior drawer test will correct this position to the normal (hence *posterior drawer sign*), thus distinguishing the signs from those of anterior cruciate rupture.

The Tibiofibular Joint

The tibia and fibula are connected at their upper and lower ends by joints—the *superior* and *inferior tibiofibular* joints—and their shafts are joined by the crural *interosseus membrane*.

The superior tibiofibular joint

This is a plane joint with flat oval articular surfaces (facets) between the lateral condyle of the tibia and the fibular head.

The *capsular ligament* attaches to the margins of the facets and is much thicker *anteriorly*. The synovial membrane of the joint may in some cases communicate with the knee joint through the popliteal bursa. The *anterior ligament* is two or three flat bands passing from the front of the fibular head obliquely upwards to the front of the lateral tibial condyle. The *posterior ligament* is a thick band from the back of the fibular head passing upwards obliquely to posterior aspect of lateral tibial condyle.

The *anterior tibial vessels* pass between the tibia and fibula, through a gap in the upper interosseous membrane just below the fibular head.

The *lateral popliteal nerve* follows a line drawn from the apex of the popliteal fossa downwards and laterally along the medial side of the biceps tendon to the posterior head of the fibula—*it can be rolled against the bone at this site*. It lies between the biceps femoris tendon and lateral head of gastrocnemius, winding around the fibular neck deep to the peroneus longus. and then divides into musculocutaneous and anterior tibial nerves.

Examination

Look for swelling by observing any difference between the two sides in the contour of the lateral aspects below the joint. This is best observed from *above* with the knees *flexed*.

Palpate the joint-line for tenderness and then assess laxity by flexing the knee to about 85° and then pulling forward with three fingers pressing forward on the head and neck of the fibula. Note any sensory symptoms produced by these manœuvres or by tapping the back of the fibular head (Tinel's test), indicating irritation of the lateral popliteal nerve.

Local Aspiration and Injection

Arthrocentesis of the knee joint

There are four major entry sites suitable for knee aspiration, medial retropatellar, lateral retropatellar, suprapatellar and anterior. Whatever the approach used, corticosteroids should only be injected into the joint if a clear diagnosis which justifies injection has been made. A strict aseptic technique is essential for any aspiration.

The knee is the easiest joint to enter and, since it is commonly affected by inflammatory joint disease and noninflammatory effusions, it is the joint most frequently aspirated as a means of both diagnosis and treatment. The large capacity of the joint and the very large synovial surface area may result in huge effusions, but also a significant absorption of corticosteroid when injected into the joint, which may result in sufficient blood levels to produce a systemic 'steroid boost' effect. Aspiration to dryness may in itself give considerable pain relief and, where a large popliteal cyst has formed, removal of the fluid, allowing decompression of the cyst, may allow the knee to regain full extension.

Medial retropatellar approach

The medial approach is the easiest when there is a moderate or large effusion. This is performed with the patient lying supine on a firm couch with the lower limbs extended. It is essential to encourage the patient to relax, so that the quadriceps muscle is not tensed as this will clamp the patella down into the patellar groove, blocking needle introduction.

The site of entry medially (Fig. 17) is just below the midpoint of the patella. The needle is introduced in a line towards the suprapatellar pouch. It is important to aspirate back as the needle is progressed, as fluid may be found after/above only 1.5 cm of penetration. In this way, too deep introduction of the needle, with possible damage to the articular cartilage, will be avoided.

As the fluid is aspirated it can be 'milked down' by controlled pressure with one hand over the suprapatellar pouch.

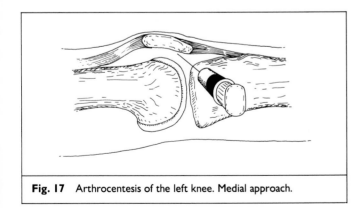

Fig. 17 Arthrocentesis of the left knee. Medial approach.

Lateral retropatellar approach

The patient should lie flat and supine with the knee extended. The line of injection is at the point of the

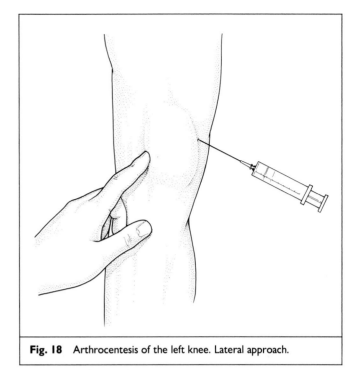

Fig. 18 Arthrocentesis of the left knee. Lateral approach.

junction of the middle and upper thirds of the patella (Fig. 18). One hand can be placed on the inner aspect of the patella and used to slightly displace the patella laterally, which increases the gap between patella and femur laterally. The needle (21 gauge is usually sufficient) should be introduced at the junction point described above, upwards towards the suprapatellar pouch. As the needle is introduced, aspiration back should be performed and this will prevent pushing the needle too far (which usually means introduction into fatty tissue behind the suprapatellar pouch).

Suprapatellar approach

If there is a very large effusion, expanding the suprapatellar bursa, the needle can be introduced into the suprapatellar pouch above and just lateral to the patella.

Anterior approach

An anterior approach, with the knee flexed to 90°, was favoured by some clinicians as it avoided the risk of needling articular cartilage, but it is rarely used now.

The needle is inserted just below the patella pole and to the side of the patellar tendon. It is introduced parallel to the line of the tibial plateau, entering the intercondylar fossa between the medial and lateral condyles after 4–5 cm.

Corticosteroid injection

Where a clear diagnosis meriting corticosteroid injection has been made, a long-acting preparation, such as triamcinolone hexacetonide or methylprednisolone acetate, should be introduced. The patient should be advised to reduce walking and knee exercising for the immediate 24–48 h period after injection, to reduce systemic absorption of the drug.

Soft-tissue injection around the knee

Many painful soft-tissue conditions around the knee respond to local corticosteroid injection. However, a clear indication for injection must be confirmed and accurate anatomical localisation of the injection defined.

The most common conditions requiring injection and their localisation are described below. They are all best injected using a short-acting preparation (hydrocortisone acetate 25.0–37.5 mg) mixed with a small volume of lignocaine, provided there is no history of previous allergic reaction.

Bursitis

It is essential that, if an infected bursa is suspected (usually prepatellar), the needle is *not* introduced into the knee joint itself, as this carries the risk of spreading infection into the joint. Even in a septic bursitis, fluid may not be obtained, but a small volume of local anaesthetic or sterile saline can be injected and then aspirated back to provide a specimen for culture.

The *prepatellar bursa* (Fig. 19) should be injected towards the centre of the maximum point of fluctuance, usually over or just below the lower portion of the patella, with the needle at an angle of about 30° to the skin.

The *deep infrapatellar bursa* should be approached from either the medial or lateral aspect and the needle directed deep to the patellar ligament, proximal to its insertion to the tibial tubercle. This may be enlarged due to Osgood–Schlatter's disease previously with calcific debris behind the ligament irritating this and the bursa. Frequent recurrence despite injection should be treated surgically.

Attachment lesions in osteoarthritis of the knee

In osteoarthritis of the knee, pain is commonly localised to one of the collateral ligament attachments (usually the medial), and may be elicited by stress testing or by finding tenderness by pressing with one finger over the attachment (Fig. 20). Infiltration of the tender area with hydrocortisone is often very helpful, provided there is no major instability.

In patellofemoral osteoarthritis, persistent and localised tender sites in the patellar retinaculum attachment to the patellar borders may respond to local injection, but the needle should not enter the joint. These tender sites must be localised accurately by displacing the patella with one hand and then palpating the patellar edge on the opposite side with one finger (Fig. 21). A tender *medial plica*, which can be

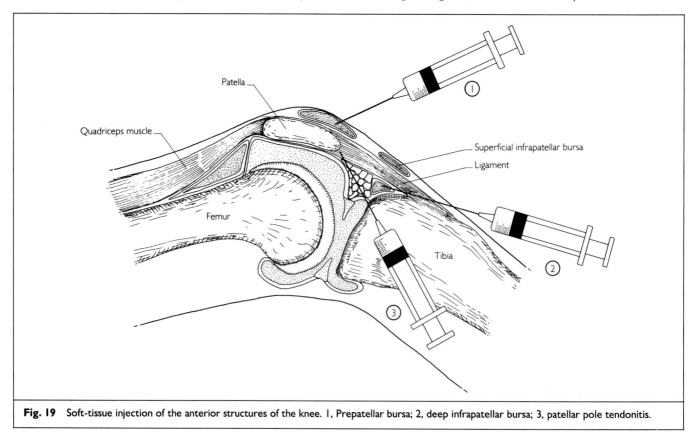

Fig. 19 Soft-tissue injection of the anterior structures of the knee. 1, Prepatellar bursa; 2, deep infrapatellar bursa; 3, patellar pole tendonitis.

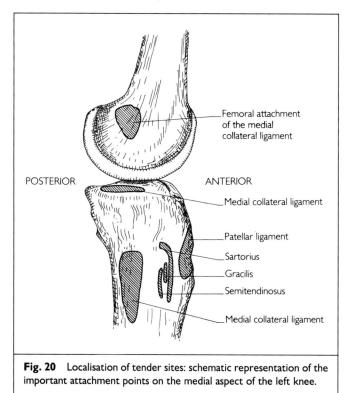

Fig. 20 Localisation of tender sites: schematic representation of the important attachment points on the medial aspect of the left knee.

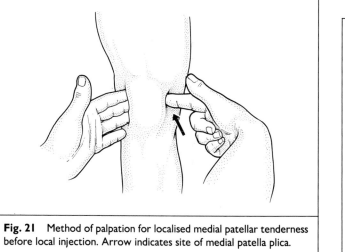

Fig. 21 Method of palpation for localised medial patellar tenderness before local injection. Arrow indicates site of medial patella plica.

rolled under the finger at about the midpoint of the medial aspect of the patella, should be excluded in the athlete.

Tendinitis

Chronic inflammation at the attachment of the patellar tendon (ligament) to the inferior patellar pole, and less commonly the superior patellar pole, usually responds well to local injection, provided there is no deep-seated necrotic tendon lesion, with extension of tenderness down the patellar tendon. These more serious tendon lesions can be confirmed by ultrasound, computerised tomography or nuclear magnetic resonance scanning and may require surgical intervention.

The *inferior patellar attachment* should be injected (Fig. 19) by accurately localising the maximal point of tenderness and then by directing the needle, after insertion just to the side of the tendon, at an angle of about 45°, with the knee extended so that the posterior attachment is infiltrated together with the paratendon as the needle is withdrawn. About 7 days after injection a graduated restrengthening programme of quadriceps exercises must be followed as full recovery of tendon strength takes many months.

Iliotibial band syndrome

Injection should be directed towards the most tender site, which is most commonly where the iliotibial band slips backwards and forwards over the lateral femoral condyle as the knee flexes and extends, particularly in distance road runners (especially camber running). There may be swelling due to a burstis under the iliotibial band which should be injected (Fig. 22).

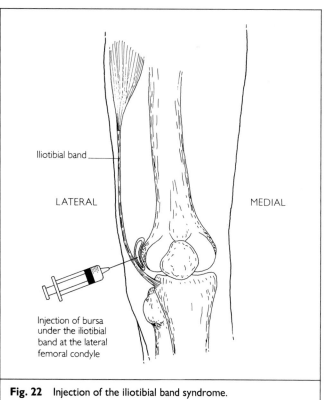

Fig. 22 Injection of the iliotibial band syndrome.

7

THE FOOT AND ANKLE

The foot and ankle are specially designed to transmit body weight. The joints are capable of adjusting to cope with various terrains and the thick heel and toe pads are designed as 'shock absorbers'. In addition to being targets for systemic arthropathies, because of concentrated stresses, the foot and ankle often develop static deformities.

Anatomy

The joints (Figs 1 and 2)

The distal tibiofibular joint
This is a fibrous joint which allows slight separation during ankle dorsiflexion. It is strengthened by anterior and posterior ligaments and a deep transverse tibiofibular ligament.

The ankle joint (talocrural)
This is a hinge joint between the distal tibia and fibula and the trochlear of the talus. The medial and lateral malleoli project distally to form a mortise that holds the talus preventing rotation or lateral flexion. The tibia in fact forms the weight-bearing portion of the ankle joint and the axis of movement passes through

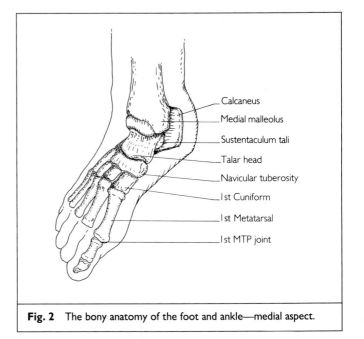

Fig. 2   The bony anatomy of the foot and ankle—medial aspect.

the malleoli. The trochlea of the talus is wider anteriorly than posteriorly. Therefore the ankle is more stable in dorsiflexion, as in ascending inclines, than in plantar flexion, as in descending. The joint capsule is attached around the articular margins of the tibia, fibula and talus. It is lax and weak on the anterior and posterior aspects of the ankle and anteriorly it is particularly extensive extending from the tibia to a point approximately 1 cm distal to the neck of the talus. The capsule is lined by synovium, and the articular cavity does not communicate with other joints or bursae. At the sides, the joint is strengthened by collateral ligaments (Fig. 3). The lateral collateral ligament is in three distinct bands each of which can be separately damaged in a sprain injury. The medial (deltoid) ligament is triangular shaped joining the medial malleolus to the talus, navicular and calcaneus. It is stronger than the lateral ligament, and during eversion injury, rather than ligament rupture, the medial malleolus is fractured.

The intertarsal joints
The foot has three functional units, the hindfoot comprising the calcaneus and talus, the midfoot

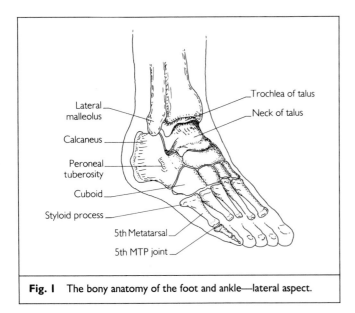

Fig. 1   The bony anatomy of the foot and ankle—lateral aspect.

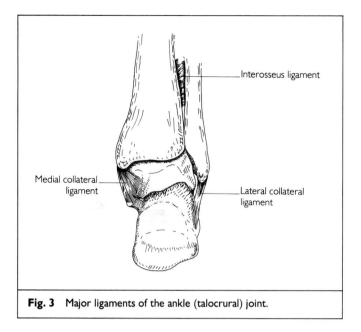

Fig. 3 Major ligaments of the ankle (talocrural) joint.

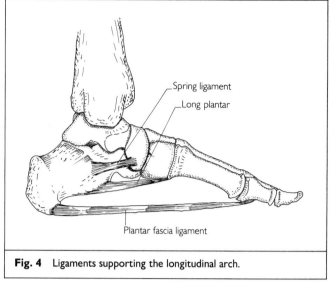

Fig. 4 Ligaments supporting the longitudinal arch.

comprising five small tarsal bones, and the forefoot consisting of the metatarsals and phalanges. The *subtalar (talocalcaneal) joint* is between the concave facet on the upper surface of the talus and the posterior convex facet on the upper surface of the calcaneus. It is sometimes known as the posterior subtalar joint. It permits inversion and eversion of the foot allowing one to stand upright on a sloping surface. The *midtarsal joint* is a composite formed by the *talocalcaneonavicular* joint and the *calcaneocuboid* joint. It allows the forefoot to invert (supinate) and evert (pronate) on the midfoot and other intertarsal joints and the tarsometatarsal joints add to the movement. The *talocalcaneonavicular joint* is a ball-and-socket joint between the head of the talus and a socket formed by the concave posterior surface of the navicular and anterior facet in the upper surface of the calcaneus (sometimes known as the anterior subtalar joint).

The metatarsophalangeal joints and interphalangeal joints

These are ellipsoid joints similar to the metacarpophalangeal joints of the hand. Each joint has a thick plantar (volar) plate, the plates being connected by the deep transverse metatarsal ligament. Two sesamoid bones are embedded into the volar plate beneath the hallux. The joints are flexed by the intrinsic muscles of the foot, while the extensor hallucis longus and extensor digitorum longus and brevis are dorsiflexors.
The interphalangeal joints are hinge joints which flex during the push-off phase of gait. In addition to helping to provide leverage for propelling the body forwards, the toes also provide stability and balance in both standing and movement by their gripping action on the ground.

The arch of the foot

This enables the weight of the body to be equally distributed between the posterior part of the calcaneus, which forms the prominence of the heel, and the heads of the four metatarsals and the two sesamoids of the first metatarsal anteriorly. The basic structure of the arch, which has a longitudinal and transverse component, is provided by the shape of the small bones of the foot united by many articular joints and supported by ligaments and muscles to provide flexibility and spring to facilitate walking and running.

The longitudinal arch is high and flexible on the medial side where it is formed by the medial three metatarsals, cuneiforms, navicular, talus and calcaneus. It is supported by several layers of ligaments (Fig. 4). Deepest is the strong spring ligament (plantar calcaneonavicular ligament), a broad thick band which connects the medial projection of the calcaneus (sustentaculum tali) to the navicular. Then the long and short plantar ligaments join the calcaneus to the metatarsal bones and the cuboid. The most superficial layer is the plantar fascia which extends from the posterior inferior surface of the calcaneus to the transverse metatarsal ligament and the flexor tendon sheath of the toes, and acts as a strong tie between the weight-bearing points of the foot. The lateral side of the longitudinal arch is low and rigid. The transverse arch is highest proximally across the cuboid and cuneiforms, and low distally across the metatarsal necks.

Tendons and bursae

Anterior to the ankle are three tendon sheaths held in place by the extensor retinaculum (Fig. 5). This consists of a superior part (transverse crural ligament) in

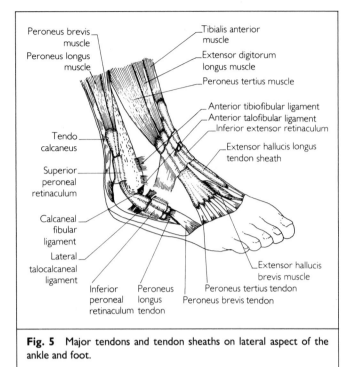

Fig. 5 Major tendons and tendon sheaths on lateral aspect of the ankle and foot.

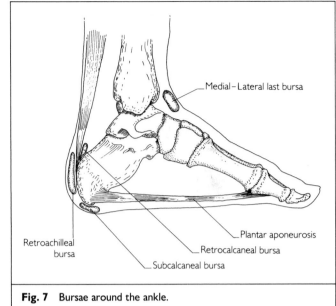

Fig. 7 Bursae around the ankle.

the anterior and inferior portion of the leg and an inferior part (cruciate ligament) in the proximal portion of the dorsum of the foot. The medial tendon sheath contains the tibialis anterior, the central sheath contains the extensor hallucis longus, extensor digitorum and peroneus tertius. Behind and below the lateral malleolus are the peroneus longus and brevis held down by the peroneal retinaculum, which consists of a superior and an inferior part.

Behind and below the medial malleolus are the tendons of the tibialis posterior, flexor digitorum longus and flexor hallucis longus, each in a tendon sheath (Fig. 6). These are held in place by the flexor

retinaculum. Posteriorly the Achilles tendon (tendo calcaneus), the common tendon of the gastrocnemius and soleus, is inserted into the posterior aspect of the calcaneus. There are bursae between the skin and the Achilles tendon, and between the tendon and the calcaneus (Fig. 7). There is also a small bursa anterior to the medial and lateral malleolus.

The tarsal tunnel lies between the medial malleolus and the calcaneus, roofed by the flexor retinaculum. In addition to tendons, the posterior tibial nerve passes through the tunnel.

Development

Lower limb buds first appear at about the fourth week of embryonic life. By 6–8 weeks proximal and distal segments are apparent and toes begin differentiation. Cartilaginous precursors of future bones develop. Bones of the foot are still largely cartilaginous at birth and are still deformable. Ossification occurs throughout the first 3 years and fusion of the phalangeal and metatarsal epiphyses is complete by late adolescence. The arch of the foot does not appear until approximately the third year and can be delayed until adolescence.

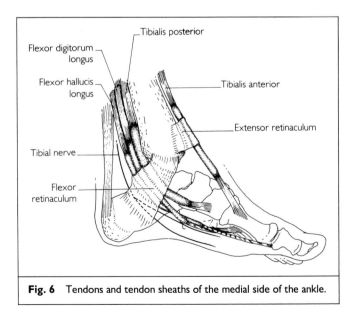

Fig. 6 Tendons and tendon sheaths of the medial side of the ankle.

Developmental abnormalities

Clubfoot (talipes) is a deformity of the ankle and foot (Fig. 8). There may be plantar flexion of the ankle (talipes equinus) or dorsiflexion (talipes calcaneus). Often there is an associated midfoot deformity, for example, talipes equinovarus or talipes calcaneovalgus.

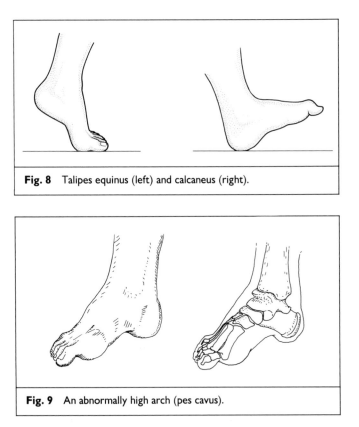

Fig. 8 Talipes equinus (left) and calcaneus (right).

Fig. 9 An abnormally high arch (pes cavus).

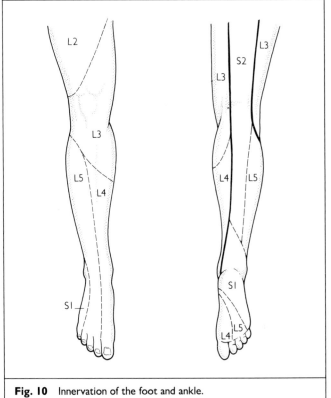

Fig. 10 Innervation of the foot and ankle.

Flat foot (pes planus) is where there is absence of a longitudinal arch. This may be associated with a valgus deformity of the midfoot. *Pes cavus* is the opposite (Fig. 9) and is often associated with a varus deformity. Abnormal fibrous, bony or cartilaginous connections between the bones of the hind- and midfoot result in tarsal coalition. It often results in a painful, pronated gait because of lack of movement between the involved bones, with spasm of adjacent muscles.

The metatarsals may be adducted. Involvement of the first metatarsal (*metatarsus primus varus*) is most common and may precede hallux valgus deformity. Toes may be shortened (*brachydactyly*), fused (*syndactyly*), decreased in number (*hypodactyly*), absent (*adactyly*) or there may be extra toes (*polydactyly*).

Symptoms

Pain is the principal symptom. In synovitis, pain is often diffuse and accompanied by prolonged stiffness, typically in the mornings. When due to static deformities, osteoarthritis and metatarsalgia, pain is more obviously associated with weight-bearing. Pain from the talocrural and the subtalar joints arises from the ankle and is aggravated by standing or walking, particularly on uneven terrain in the case of the subtalar joints. With the midtarsal joints pain is felt midway down the foot, while in the case of the MTP joints

there is a characteristic sensation of 'walking on marbles', with pain localised to the metatarsal heads. Burning pain in the soles and toes may be caused by plantar neuralgia, Morton's neuroma (which often causes burning pain between the 3rd and 4th digits) and a tarsal tunnel syndrome.

The innervation of the foot is shown in Figure 10. The spine and all the other lower extremity joints should be examined, since pathology of these sites can be the cause of pain referred to the foot and ankle.

Referred pain from irritation of the first sacral nerve root affects the heel and the lateral side of the foot, is exacerbated by straight-leg raising, and may be accompanied by other neurological signs.

Tarsal tunnel syndrome

This is caused by entrapment of the posterior tibial nerve beneath the flexor retinaculum behind and under the medial malleolus. Symptoms of burning, tingling and numbness can be felt throughout the distribution of the posterior tibial nerve but is often most pronounced in the toes and the distal part of the sole. Often there is tenderness along the nerve at the margin of the medial malleolus, and there may be the equivalent of a Tinel's sign. Sometimes there is reduced pin-prick sensation but motor weakness and atrophy of the toe flexors and abductor hallucis is not common. Neurophysiological tests may demonstrate prolonged nerve conduction distal to the compression.

Examination

Inspection

Examination of the foot and ankle must include inspection of the whole lower limb and therefore the patient should remove clothing from the waist down. The ankle and foot are inspected both resting and standing, together with the footwear which can provide important clues. Both sides are compared from all angles for swelling, deformities, the location of calluses and bursal reactions, the presence of other cutaneous manifestations and the appearance of the nails.

Inflammation producing capsular distension of the ankle joint produces diffuse swelling anteriorly, which obliterates the small depressions normally present in front of the malleoli. Sometimes there is swelling in the area of the tarsal tunnel just posterior to the joint between the malleoli and the Achilles tendon. Swelling of the ankle may be accentuated by dorsiflexion and inversion of the foot, which produces bulging beneath the extensor tendons in front of the lateral and medial malleolar ligaments.

Capsular distension of the midtarsal joint is less common but can produce diffuse swelling over the dorsum of the hindfoot. The MTP joints, however, frequently become swollen, being apparent in the dorsum of the forefoot and obscuring the visibility of the extensor tendons. Associated inflammation of ligaments bracing the forefoot results in spreading the metatarsals and toes.

Tenosynovitis of ankle extensors produces linear swelling across the ankle joint. Digital flexor tenosynovitis produces 'sausage' toes, which are characteristic of psoriatic arthritis.

In oedematous states, fluid collects below and behind the malleoli where tissues are most lax, producing swelling that pits.

In pes planus or flat foot there is loss of the longitudinal arch. In extreme cases the translocated talus and navicula produce a prominence in front of and slightly below the medial malleolus. The converse is pes cavus, which is mostly the result of neurological disease such as spina bifida and cerebellar ataxia. Fixed plantar flexion of the foot (talipes equinus) is usually the result of spastic paralysis but can occur in rheumatoid arthritis as a result of shortening of the Achilles. Deformities of the subtalar joint, calcaneovalgus (eversion) or calcaneovarus (inversion) are best observed from the back.

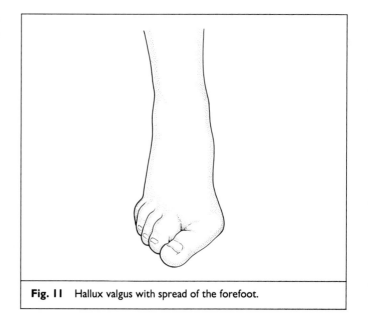

Fig. 11 Hallux valgus with spread of the forefoot.

The commonest deformity of the big toe is hallux valgus (Fig. 11). There is lateral deviation of the big toe as a result of abnormal angulation and rotation of the first MTP joint. The first metatarsal deviates medially, resulting in increased width of the forefoot. Frequently there is a bursal reaction resulting in a bunion over the medial aspect of the joint. A hammer toe deformity (Fig. 12) results from hyperextension of the MTP joint, flexion of the proximal interphalangeal joint (PIP) and hyperextension of the distal interphalangeal joint (DIP). A callus often develops over the prominent PIP joint. The second toe is most often affected and this is frequently associated with hallux valgus of the big toe. This may occur with or without arthritis as an underlying cause. Sometimes the DIP is

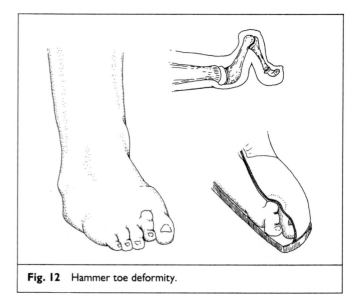

Fig. 12 Hammer toe deformity.

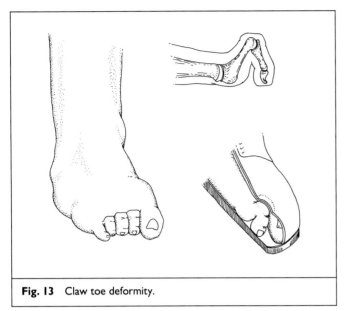

Fig. 13 Claw toe deformity.

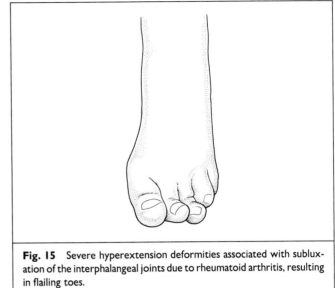

Fig. 15 Severe hyperextension deformities associated with subluxation of the interphalangeal joints due to rheumatoid arthritis, resulting in flailing toes.

in a neutral position so that the tip of the toe touches the floor. This is a 'mallet toe'.

Cock-up (or claw) toe deformities (Fig. 13) are the result of flexion of the interphalangeal joints secondary to plantar subluxation of the MTP joints. There is often callus formation on the sole over the metatarsal heads and metatarsal spread due to weakening of the transverse metatarsal ligament. This is associated with a polyarthritis such as rheumatoid arthritis. Severe articular damage of the interphalangeal joints results in hyperextension deformities of the toes. Also there can be lateral displacement of the proximal phalanges on the metatarsal head of all the toes, equivalent to 'ulnar deviation' of the fingers, leading to overlapping of the toes (Figs 14 and 15).

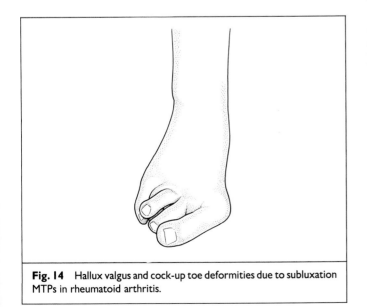

Fig. 14 Hallux valgus and cock-up toe deformities due to subluxation MTPs in rheumatoid arthritis.

Abnormalities of gait may be observed. These include the toe-out gait, with outward displacement of the forefoot and an attempt to walk by rolling the foot from the lateral to the medial side. This happens in patients with painful ankles and often results in an eversion deformity and loss of the longitudinal arch so that the patient walks on the medial aspect of the foot. A toe-in gait (pigeon-toe) is due to inward displacement of the forefoot which is often congenital and associated with inversion of the foot. Those with a painful heel will not allow the heel to strike the ground, and a foot drop results in a typical 'slap' of the foot on the ground.

When examining the shoes, a broken medial counter is typical of flat feet, excessive wear of the lateral border of the shoe is typical of hallux rigidus and scuffed toes occur in those with a dropped foot.

In addition to defining calluses, examination of the skin and nails may demonstrate psoriasis or other characteristic lesions such as keratoderma blenorrhagica. Dependent rubor indicates vascular disease.

Palpation

The examiner is best facing the patient who sits on the edge of the couch with the legs dangling free. With one hand cupping the heel to support the foot, the examiner palpates the anterior aspect of the ankle and forefoot with the fingers (Fig. 16) or thumb (Fig. 17) of the other hand. An alternative method is to support the foot with the fingers of both hands and use both thumbs to palpate the tissue anteriorly (Fig. 18). Since synovial reflection is most extensive over the anterior aspect of the joint, synovial thickening or effusion is likely to be palpable anteriorly. Sometimes it is best palpated medially and laterally between the extensor

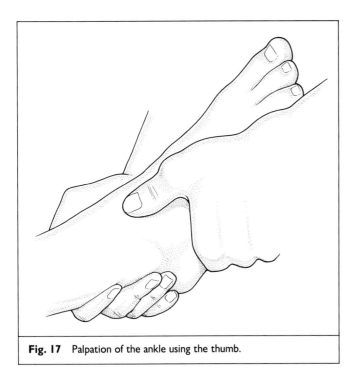

Fig. 16 Palpation of the ankle. The patient's foot is supported by the examiner's hand which compresses the posterior aspect of the articular capsule. This distends the articular capsule and synovial membrane anteriorly, where they can be palpated by the fingers of the examiner's hand.

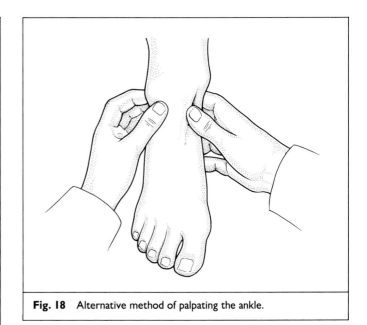

Fig. 18 Alternative method of palpating the ankle.

the joint-line medial to the tendon of tibialis anterior (the most medial of the three extensor tendons). Tenosynovitis overlying the anterior aspect of the ankle joint can be distinguished from underlying synovitis by more superficial linear swelling and tenderness, which extends beyond the joint margin, over the distribution of the tendon sheaths. Pain produced by resisted movement of the affected tendon is also characteristic.

The subtalar joint is not accessible to palpation but the intertarsal joints can be palpated for swelling and tenderness, which is mainly detected in the dorsum of the foot. The head of the talus becomes prominent on the medial side of the foot in pes planus (Fig. 19), and

Fig. 17 Palpation of the ankle using the thumb.

retinaculum and malleoli. By compressing the area beneath and behind the medial and lateral malleoli with the supporting hand, thus compressing the posterior aspect of the articular capsule, the anterior capsule can be distended with synovial fluid. The anterior capsule is best palpated for tenderness over

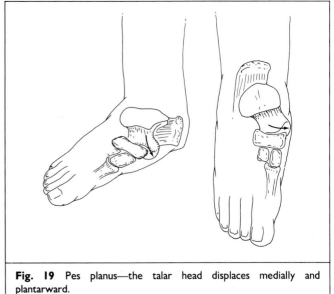

Fig. 19 Pes planus—the talar head displaces medially and plantarward.

there may be overlying tenderness and callus from pressing against the shoe (Fig. 20). In children there may be tenderness over the navicular tubercle as a result of osteonecrosis (Fig. 21).

The MTP joints are palpated between the examiner's thumbs on the dorsum of the foot, and the forefinger on the plantar aspect over the metatarsal head. Each joint is examined individually for soft-tissue thickening, deformity and tenderness (Fig. 22). The medial aspect of the first MTP is a common site for a tender and inflamed bursa (Fig. 23). It is also a common site for tophi. In the presence of chronic synovitis, there is frequently subluxation of the MTP joints with dorsal displacement of the proximal pha-

lanx and loss of the normal fat pad under the metatarsal bones so that the metatarsal heads are easily palpated. Synovial proliferation and joint effusion can be palpated as soft-tissue thickening partially obliterating the grooves between adjacent metatarsal heads. Sometimes tenderness over specific joints

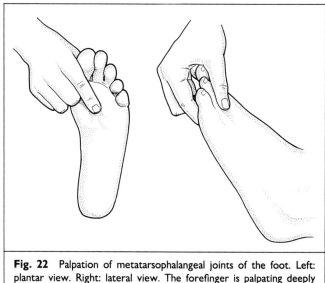

Fig. 22 Palpation of metatarsophalangeal joints of the foot. Left: plantar view. Right: lateral view. The forefinger is palpating deeply between the second and third metatarsal head.

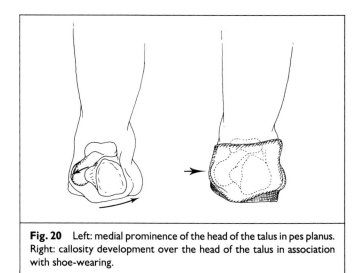

Fig. 20 Left: medial prominence of the head of the talus in pes planus. Right: callosity development over the head of the talus in association with shoe-wearing.

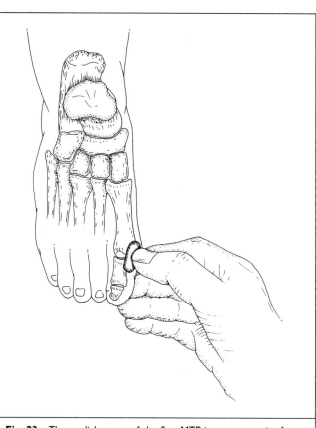

Fig. 21 The navicular tubercle (arrow).

Fig. 23 The medial aspect of the first MTP is a common site for an inflamed bursa.

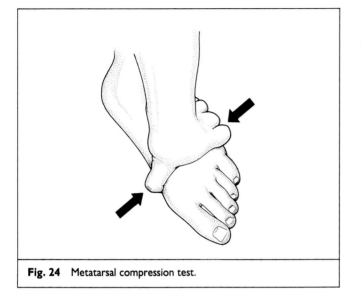

Fig. 24 Metatarsal compression test.

cannot be elicited but this important sign of synovitis may be obtained by grasping the forefoot and squeezing the metatarsal heads together between the thumb on one side of the foot and the fingers on the other (the metatarsal compression test—Fig 24).

Sharply localised tenderness between the 3rd and 4th (less commonly between the 2nd and 3rd) metatarsal heads is characteristic of Morton's interdigital neuroma. Tenderness may be accompanied by altered sensation on the lateral and medial aspects of the 3rd and 4th toes, respectively and, very occasionally, a large interdigital neuroma may be palpated. Localised

tenderness over the dorsum of the 2nd or 3rd metatarsal (although any metatarsal can be involved) may indicate a 'march' fracture.

The thumb and forefinger are used to palpate the interphalangeal joints of the toes. Swelling and tenderness due to synovitis are most prominent on the medial and lateral aspects of the joint. The Achilles tendon is palpated between thumb and forefinger for swelling, tenderness and the presence of nodules such as rheumatoid nodules, xanthomata or tophi. There are both local and systemic causes of tenosynovitis of the Achilles tendon, and these may also cause inflammation of related structures. The calcaneal bursa, for example, lying between the skin and the insertion of the Achilles tendon, is particularly subject to local trauma (Fig. 25). On the other hand, inflammation of the deeper retrocalcaneal bursa between the calcaneus and the Achilles tendon may signify inflammation due to a systemic cause. After rupture of the Achilles tendon, a defect may be palpable. To test the continuity of the tendon, the patient lies prone on the couch. On squeezing the calf, the normal plantar flexion of the foot is greatly reduced or absent after rupture of the tendon (Fig. 26).

The plantar surface of the foot should be smooth and non-tender. Tenderness on the sole near the heel may indicate plantar fasciitis, which may be the result of local trauma of part of a systemic disorder. Sometimes the tenderness arises from soft tissues overlying a bony spur on the plantar surface of the calcaneum, near the site of attachment of the plantar fascia (Fig. 27).

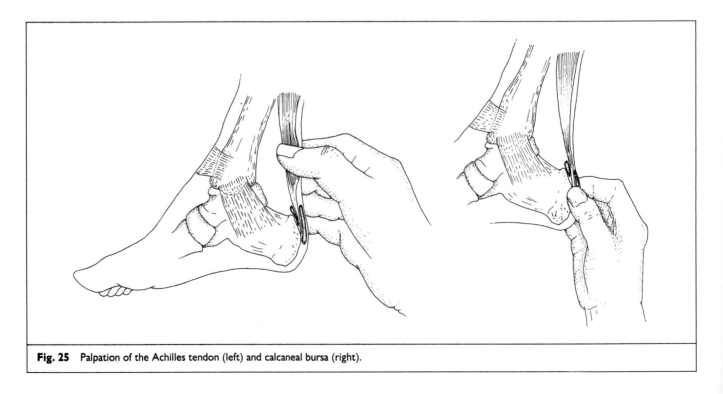

Fig. 25 Palpation of the Achilles tendon (left) and calcaneal bursa (right).

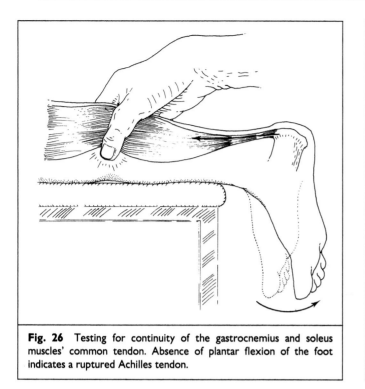

Fig. 26 Testing for continuity of the gastrocnemius and soleus muscles' common tendon. Absence of plantar flexion of the foot indicates a ruptured Achilles tendon.

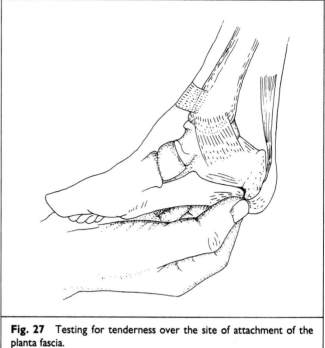

Fig. 27 Testing for tenderness over the site of attachment of the planta fascia.

Range of movements

Figure 28 illustrates techniques to screen for gross restriction of ankle and foot movement. These should be followed by more detailed examination of the passive range of movements.

Ankles

Movements should be tested with the knees flexed and the legs dangling to relax the gastrocnemius. Stabilise the subtalar joint by grasping the calcaneum, and avoid forefoot movement by inverting the forefoot and pushing the foot as one unit with the examiner's other hand into dorsiflexion and plantar flexion (Fig. 29). In the damaged joint the movement is restricted, painful and often accompanied by crepitus. In synovitis, the range is restricted and the extremes of dorsiflexion and plantar flexion are painful. Restricted movement may also be due to periarticular oedema from various causes and contraction of the joint capsule and periarticular tissues.

To examine movements of the subtalar joint, stabilise the distal leg with one hand and grasp the heel with the other to move the foot into inversion and eversion (Fig. 30). Movement of the midtarsal joint is tested by holding the calcaneum in one hand and rotating the foot with the other in the plane of the sole of the foot (Fig. 31, showing 30° inversion and 40° eversion). Figure 32 shows the range of flexion and extension in the 1st MTP. The other MTP joints have approximately 40° of flexion and extension. The PIP joints flex to approximately 50°, and the DIPs to approximately 40° with a varying degree of extension up to 30°.

Tests of stability

The anterior drawer signs tests the integrity of the anterior talofibular ligament (Fig. 33). Placing one

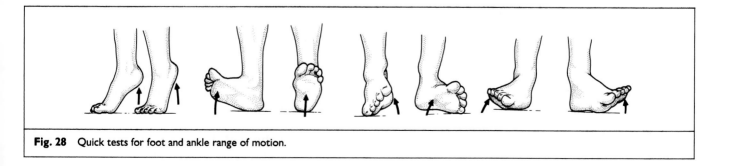

Fig. 28 Quick tests for foot and ankle range of motion.

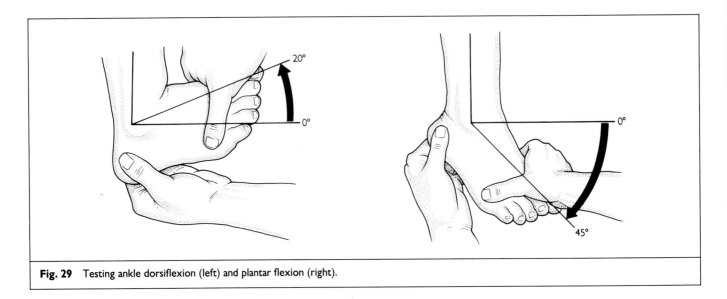

Fig. 29 Testing ankle dorsiflexion (left) and plantar flexion (right).

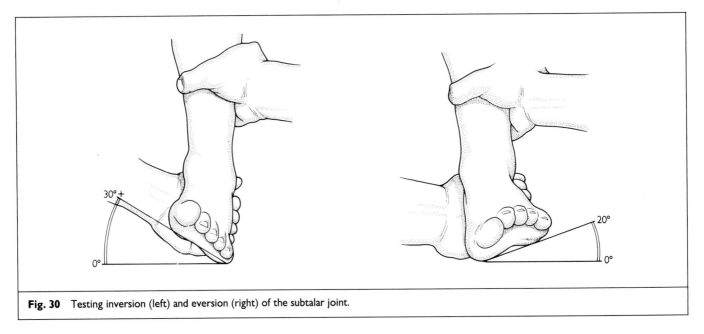

Fig. 30 Testing inversion (left) and eversion (right) of the subtalar joint.

hand on the anterior aspect of the lower tibia, the examiner grasps the calcaneus with the other hand and draws the calcaneus and talus anteriorly while pushing the tibia posteriorly. Movement, which is normally not present, indicates tear of the ligament usually as a result of a severe sprain. To test for lateral instability, which results from damage to both the anterior talofibular ligament and the calcaneofibular ligament, invert the calcaneus. On the lateral side a 'gap' appears between the talus and the calcaneus (Fig. 34). For deltoid ligament insufficiency the calcaneus is everted and a gap develops between the talus and calcaneum.

Muscle testing (Table 1)

Plantar flexion. Unless there is major foot deformity,

inability of the patient to walk on toes indicates significant muscle weakness. Gross muscle weakness can also be assessed when the patient lies supine with legs extended and a pad under the knees to prevent hyperextension. Stabilising the lower leg with one hand, the examiner's other hand provides graded resistance to plantar flexion (Fig. 35).

Dorsiflexion and inversion. If the patient can walk on his or her heels, muscle strength is considered normal. Alternatively, test the tibialis anterior with the patient sitting, using one hand to stabilise the lower leg and the other to provide resistance to flexion and inversion (Fig. 36).

Eversion of the foot. If the patient is able to walk on the medial borders of the feet, muscle strength is

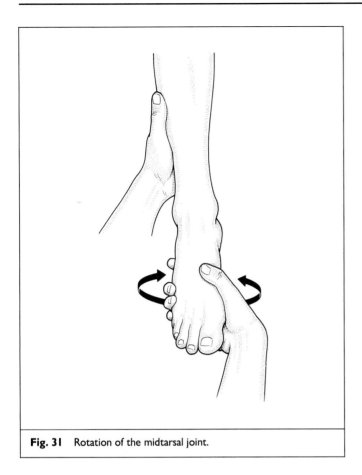

Fig. 31   Rotation of the midtarsal joint.

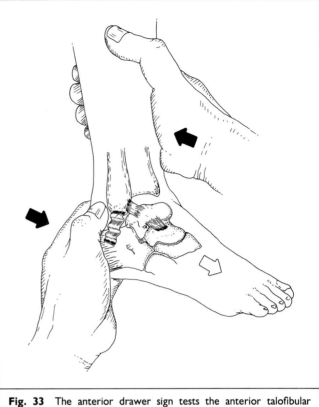

Fig. 33   The anterior drawer sign tests the anterior talofibular ligament. Movement indicates a tear of the ligament.

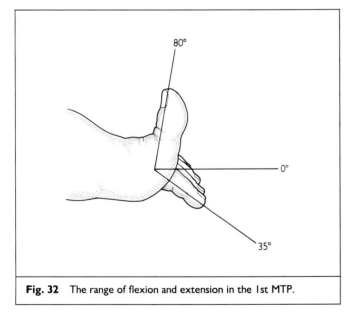

Fig. 32   The range of flexion and extension in the 1st MTP.

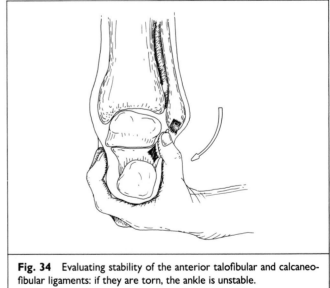

Fig. 34   Evaluating stability of the anterior talofibular and calcaneo-fibular ligaments: if they are torn, the ankle is unstable.

normal. It can be tested manually by stabilising the foot and resisting plantar flexion and eversion by pushing against the lateral border of the foot (Fig. 37).

Inversion of the foot. The tibialis posterior is tested by stabilising the lower leg with one hand and having the

patient plantar flex and invert the foot while the examiner resists this movement with the other hand.

Flexion and extension of the toes. To test flexion and extension of the big toe, the foot is stabilised with one hand in the midtarsal region and flexion at the MTP

Table 1. Nerve roots, peripheral nerves and muscles involved in movement of the ankle and foot

Movement	Nerve root	Peripheral nerve	Muscles
Plantar flexion	S1 S2	Tibial	Gastrocnemius, soleus (accessory muscles: tibialis posterior, peroneus longus and brevis, flexor hallucis longus, flexor digitorum longus, plantaris)
Dorsiflexion and inversion	L4 L5	Deep peroneal	Tibialis anterior
Inversion (in plantar flexion)	L5 S1	Tibial	Tibialis posterior
Eversion	S1	Superficial peroneal	Peroneus longus and brevis
Flexion of big toe			
MTP joint	L4 L5 S1	Medial plantar	Flexor hallucis brevis
IP joint	L5 S1 S2	Tibial nerve	Flexor hallucis longus
Extension of big toe			
MTP joint	L5 S1	Deep peroneal	Extensor digitorum brevis
IP joint	L4 L5 S1	Deep peroneal	Extensor hallucis longus
Flexion of toes 2–5			
MTP joint	L4 L5	Medial (1st lumbrical)	Lumbricals
	S1 S2	Lateral (2nd to 4th lumbricals) plantar	
PIP joint	L4 L5	Medial plantar	Flexor digitorum brevis
DIP joint	L5 S1	Tibial	Flexor digitorum longus
Extension of toes 2–5	L4 L5 S1	Deep peroneal	Extensor digitorum longus
	L5 S1	Deep peroneal	Extensor digitorum brevis

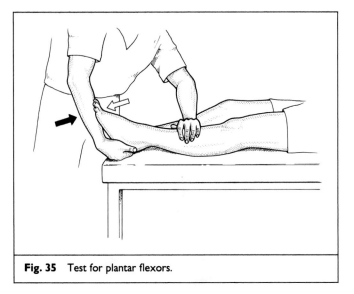
Fig. 35   Test for plantar flexors.

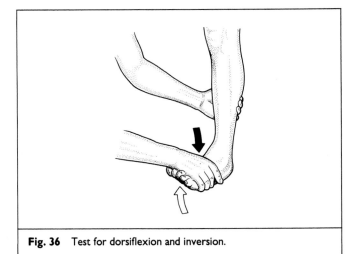
Fig. 36   Test for dorsiflexion and inversion.

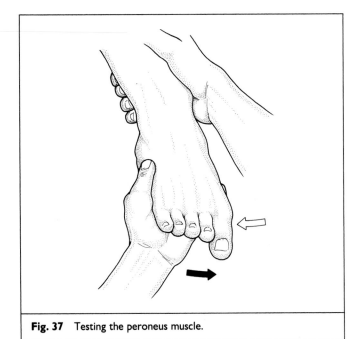
Fig. 37   Testing the peroneus muscle.

and the IP joints are assessed against resistance provided by the examiner's other hand placed beneath the proximal phalanx. Extension is tested against resistance of the examiner's thumb on the nailbed with fingers on the ball of the foot to stabilise the metatarsal. To test the extensor hallucis longus, resistance must be applied distal to the IP joint.

To test the flexors of the other toes, the patient flexes

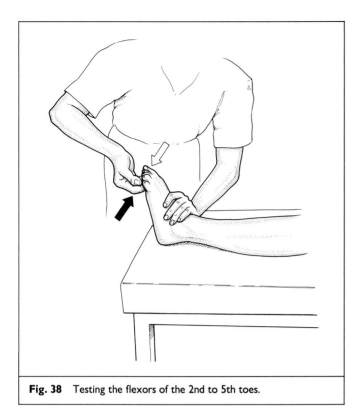

Fig. 38 Testing the flexors of the 2nd to 5th toes.

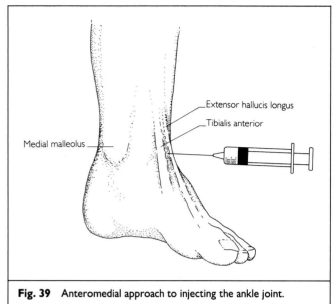

Fig. 39 Anteromedial approach to injecting the ankle joint.

these joints against resistance provided by the examiner's fingers, which are beneath the proximal row of phalanges (Fig. 38). The MT and IP joints should be unyielding.

To test extension of the toes, the calcaneus is held to stabilise the foot and resistance to movement is provided by the thumb of the examiner's other hand on the dorsum of the toes. These should be unyielding.

Local Aspiration and Injection

The ankle joint

There are several approaches to aspirating and injecting the ankle joint. The anterior approach is described here. Injection of the ankle joint is more liable to be complicated by infection than other sites, perhaps because of the tendency to oedema. Therefore a careful aseptic technique is particularly important.

With the foot in moderate plantar flexion, insert the needle in the space between the tibia and talus bounded medially by the tibialis anterior tendon and laterally by extensor hallucis longus tendon (Fig. 39). It is important to direct the needle tangentially to the curve of the talus; the most common mistake is to direct the needle too much towards the heel.

Posterior subtalar joint

This often communicates with the ankle joint particularly in rheumatoid arthritis. Therefore injection speci-

fically into this joint, which can be difficult, is not often needed. The joint can be injected using a lateral approach with the patient lying prone. The landmarks (Fig. 40) are a horizontal line drawn 2.5 cm above the distal end of the lateral malleolus, and a vertical line 1.0 cm from the posterior border of the shaft of the fibula. The point where these lines cross marks the site of entry.

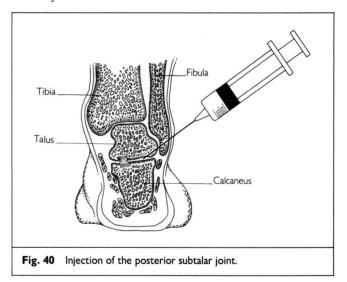

Fig. 40 Injection of the posterior subtalar joint.

Midtarsal joint

Injection is difficult. Sometimes a small-gauge needle can be inserted into an intertarsal joint space on the dorsum of the foot.

Achilles bursitis

Approach from the lateral side of the heel, just above the top of the calcaneum. Direct the needle medially and downwards into the bursa, which lies just beneath the skin. Avoid injecting the tendon *per se*.

Plantar fasciitis

Locate the site of maximum tenderness on the plantar surface of the heel. The needle can be inserted through the plantar surface or alternatively using a medial approach. Here, the needle is inserted through the thinner skin on the medial side of the heel so that the point lies beneath the tender spot, and the injection is made as close as possible to the bony surface into the tendinous insertion.

Morton's neuroma

Palpate for the point of maximum tenderness and inject.

Tenosynovitis of posterior tibial tendon

Often the tendon sheath is swollen. A tangential approach is used, directing the needle proximally. A correctly placed injection distends the tendon sheath further.

A similar procedure is used for the peroneal tendon sheaths posterior to the lateral malleolus.

Tarsal tunnel syndrome

Inject under the flexor retinaculum between the calcaneus and the medial malleolus.

8

THE TEMPOROMANDIBULAR JOINT

The articulation between mandible and cranium consists of components that are concerned with mastication, swallowing, speech and respiration, as well as mandibular posture and facial appearance. Disorders affecting the temporomandibular joints may be congenital, or arise from disease, degenerative processes, trauma or as a concomitant of occlusal stress.

Anatomy

The temporomandibular joints are unique; the mandible connects the two joints so that they move in unison—one joint cannot move alone. They are also the only joints whose movement is linked and guided by the dental occlusion, therefore tooth loss or dental restoration may affect the joints.

The primary components of the temporomandibular joint are the mandibular condyle, the articular surfaces of the temporal bone, the articular disc and the joint capsule (Fig. 1). The superior portion of the lateral pterygoid muscle is considered by some to be part of the joint because the disc is a direct extension of it; the inferior portion of the muscle attaches to the condyle. The temporomandibular joint contrasts with

other joints in that its articular surfaces are primarily composed of collagen instead of hyaline cartilage.

The disc is a dense fibrous plate that separates the joints into superior and inferior compartments. It is characterised by a thin, avascular central portion and a thicker, vascular posterior portion. The disc is normally tightly bound to the medial and lateral poles of the condyle and its main functions are stabilisation during condylar movement and shock absorption during mastication. The joint capsule attaches to the articular eminence of the temporal bone and to the condyle. The capsule is reinforced on the lateral aspect by the temporomandibular ligament, which provides some limitation to mandibular movement, and medially by the sphenomandibular ligament. The articular eminence, not the glenoid fossa, is the primary functional area of the temporal bone during mandibular movements. This is indicated by the thin bone and fibrous covering of the fossa area.

The two condylar movements during mandibular function are rotation and translation. In normal active opening of the mouth there is a combination of hinge and gliding movement. The superior joint space is associated with the anterior gliding movements of translation, whereas the inferior joint surface is associated with condylar rotation (Fig. 2). Because both temporomandibular joints are joined by a single bone, movement in one joint cannot occur without either similar co-ordinating or dissimilar reactive movements in the other joints. Opening, closing, protrusion and restriction are bilateral symmetrical movements. Lateral excursions are bilateral asymmetrical movements.

Mandibular opening is produced by contraction of the lateral pterygoid muscles with assistance from the digastric, geniohyoid, and myohyoid muscles. The masseter, medial pterygoid and anterior fibres of the temporalis muscles are involved in mandibular closing. Protrusion of the mandible is accompanied by the lateral pterygoid muscles, whereas the retruded position is produced by contraction of the posterior fibres of the temporalis muscles. Sideward movement of the mandible occurs when the contralateral lateral pterygoid muscle contracts.

The temporalis muscle plays a major role in the limitation of joint loading, and the lateral pterygoid

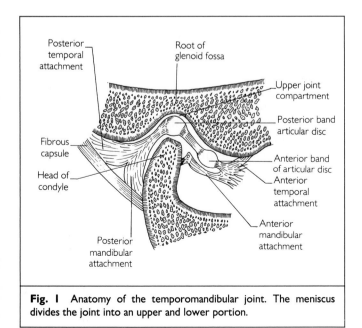

Fig. 1 Anatomy of the temporomandibular joint. The meniscus divides the joint into an upper and lower portion.

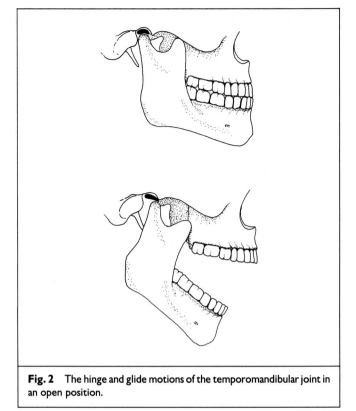

Fig. 2 The hinge and glide motions of the temporomandibular joint in an open position.

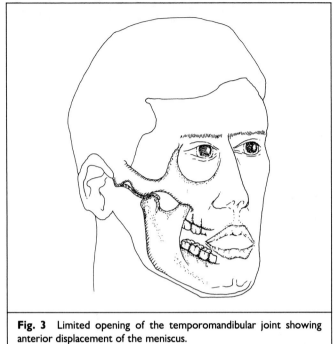

Fig. 3 Limited opening of the temporomandibular joint showing anterior displacement of the meniscus.

muscle helps to stabilise the joint by controlling both the meniscus (upper head of lateral pterygoid) and the condylar position (lower head of lateral pterygoid muscle).

The major sensory innervation of the temporomandibular joint is derived from branches of the auriculotemporal nerve, with branches of the masseteric and posterior deep temporal nerves making a smaller contribution. The capsule, lateral ligament and posterior fat pads are innervated. However, the central part of the meniscus and the synovium do not appear to be innervated.

The superficial temporal artery is the primary blood supply to the joint.

Functional Anatomy

The hinge movement of the lower joint allows some 26 mm of opening between the incisors and is seldom affected by joint dysfunction. Functional problems are usually related to the gliding or translatory movement of the upper joint space as the condyle moves forwards and down the articular eminence when the mouth opens. Restriction of opening may be a result of muscle spasm or displacement of the meniscus, which may or may not be reversible (Fig. 3).

The joint is non-load-bearing but appears to be load-bearing in some instances. This may be of importance as a cause of pain. The temporalis muscle has horizontal fibres that limit joint-loading. The aim of the conservative management of the joint (occlusal bite guards) is to reduce joint-loading and to keep the meniscus in the correct relationship to the condyle, thus restoring the dental occlusion and correcting the closing pathway determined by the interdigitation of the teeth.

Phylogenetic Development

The mammalian jaw joint is formed from membranous bones derived from the first branchial arch and cranium. In contrast, the jaw joint of most non-mammals ossifies from cartilaginous elements of the first branchial arch and its maxillary process. These primordial elements remain in the mammalian skull, but are in ossified form as the middle ear structures, malleus and incus. The articular disc, which characterises the mammalian joint, is a recent phylogenetic development.

Developmental Abnormalities

The condylar cartilage is the major mandibular growth centre, and therefore disease of the temporomandibular joint in childhood can affect mandibular development.

Familial traits of bilateral retrognathism or prognathism are not uncommon; bilateral temporomandibular maldevelopment (Treacher Collins syndrome) is very rare. Agenesis, hypoplasia or hyperplasia of the mandibular condyles, in the absence of other local or systemic anomalies, are uncommon. Severe otitis media, trauma and arthritis are the main acquired causes of impaired condylar development.

Impaired condylar growth is primarily characterised by a gradual deviation of the chin towards the affected side of the jaw, and over-eruption of teeth on the non-affected side. Bilateral involvement can cause a retrognathic 'bird-like' facial profile.

In condylar hyperplasia, there is notable bony enlargement of the affected condyle and mandibular direction towards the contralateral side.

Past Medical History

This should always be reviewed. The patient should be questioned about previous illnesses, particularly rheumatoid arthritis and degenerative joint disease. It is important to note any trauma to the head and neck. Injuries to the side of the face and chin are often responsible for temporomandibular joint problems.

The patient's dental history should also be reviewed, particularly if it coincides with the onset of symptoms.

There are numerous associated problems seen in the temporomandibular pain syndrome, and patients rarely associate these with the facial pain. Habits such as bruxism and nail biting exacerbate the pain and muscle spasm. Stress-related problems are invariably present. Tension headache with a pressure sensation over the top of the head and down the neck may be a daily occurrence. The headache may respond to simple analgesia but the dull ache in the jaw continues. Pain in the neck, back, abdomen and an irritable colon may also be present. The sleep pattern may be disturbed, and this may be marked if there is also depression.

Symptoms

Pain

Pain from the temporomandibular joint is the second most common facial pain after toothache. The main features are pain associated with mandibular movement, and often accompanied by limitation of movement. Pain can be either localised to the joint or referred to the head, neck and shoulders. The patient's description of the location, duration and characteristics of the pain greatly helps in distinguishing between disorders with similar symptoms and physical findings.

The location of the pain should be confirmed by asking the patient to indicate where it hurts. This often helps differentiate between a true joint problem, in which the patient usually localises the discomfort in the pretragos region, and a muscular discomfort. It is also important to note whether the pain is unilateral or bilateral.

Pain associated with myofascial pain dysfunction is most often described as being a dull, unilateral ache that is often worse on waking. Joint pain may be a constant, dull or sharp, but there is usually increasing discomfort with increasing function, and it is pronounced after chewing hard foods. The pain is worse on waking in many patients, but some find the pain worse at the end of the day.

Clicking

This symptom is not uncommon and may be described as 'popping' or 'snapping'; its character is quite different from crepitus, which is described as 'grating'. Clicking is usually bilateral to auscultation, but patients often think only one joint is affected. Clicking occurs at a specific point of jaw movement whereas crepitus is present throughout. Clicking may vary from day to day and be absent at times. A loss of clicking and limitation of movement indicates displacement of the meniscus. Clicking may also be eliminated by placing a spatula between the teeth simulating a bite guard.

Limitation of mandibular movement

The range of opening may be limited, this may be either constant or intermittent occurring only at the end or beginning of the day. The limitation takes the form of the jaw 'sticking' or 'locking'. Locking can vary in frequency and severity. It may occur at regular times of the day, the most common being on waking. It is sudden in onset and distressing. Patients use both terms when they have developed a way of 'freeing the joint'. This often takes the form of a lateral excursion or even pressing the mandible sideways with the hand. It may spontaneously resolve.

Locking may be a confusing term to the patient. They may describe this as jamming or dislocation of the joint. It usually occurs with the teeth slightly apart, during opening or closing of the mouth. Further movement is then prevented. Locking is the result of disc displacement. The range of movements is limited to rotational movements in the joint allowing opening to only 26 mm interincisorly, the translatory movement of the condyle and wide opening being prevented.

Examination

Inspection

Swelling of the joint must be moderate or marked before it is apparent. If swelling is detectable it appears as a rounded bulge in the area underlying the joint just anterior to the external auditory meatus.

The symmetry of the face should be assessed, although mild to moderate asymmetry is common, gross asymmetry may reflect a growth disturbance of the joint which may have resulted from trauma in childhood. Hypertrophy of the masseter muscles may indicate clenching or other oral habits.

Note the rhythm of the opening and closing of the jaw. The mandible should open and close in a straight line, with the teeth coming together and separating easily. Pathology in one or both joints or an abnormal dentition will result in abnormality.

The meniscus divides the joint cavity in two portions, an upper part used for hinge motion and a lower portion used for gliding motion. On inspection of the temporomandibular joint the two motions can be observed, the joint hinges within the glenoid fossa and glides forward to the eminentia.

Palpation

The joint can be located by placing the top of the forefinger just anterior to the external auditory meatus. On opening the mouth the top of the finger drops into an area overlying the joint. Both pretragus depressions should be palpated simultaneously. The joint can also be palpated anteriorly in the external auditory canal (Fig. 4). In the presence of synovitis the joint may be swollen and tender.

It is important to assess during pretragus and intra-auricular palpation whether the condyles move symmetrically. When unilateral problems exist, the mandible will always be seen to deviate to the side with limited condylar movement. In addition to limitation of joint movement, palpation of these areas is also used to detect clicking and crepitus. Subluxation of the joints should be noted, although it has been demonstrated to be a normal variation.

The regional muscles should be examined for tenderness and spasm. The temporalis, medial and lateral pterygoids, masseter, trapezius and sternocleidomastoid are the primary muscles included in the evaluation. The masseter muscles can be palpated bilaterally, with the fingers over the angle of the mandible. Tenderness may be detected at rest or when the jaw is clenched. The masseter muscles are most effectively examined by simultaneously pressing from inside and outside the mouth in a process of bimanual palpation.

The medial pterygoids are difficult to examine. They are checked by running a finger in an anteroposterior direction along the medial aspect of the mandible in the floor of the mouth. This can produce a gag reflex. The posterior border can be palpated extraorally by placing the fingers around the posterior border of the ramus of the mandible (Fig. 5).

The lateral pterygoid muscle is tested by placing a finger between the buccal mucosa and the superior gum and pointing the finger past the last upper molar to the neck of the mandible (Fig. 6). As the mouth opens, the neck of the mandible swings forward and the lateral pterygoid tightens. If the muscle has been damaged or is in spasm, the patient feels pain or tenderness. This muscle can also be examined by standing behind the patient, placing the palm of the hand over the chin and asking the patient to open

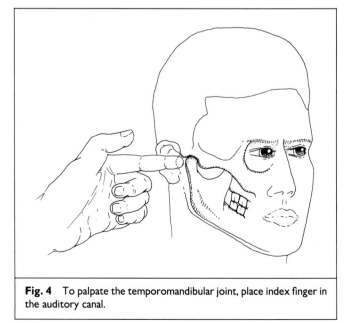

Fig. 4   To palpate the temporomandibular joint, place index finger in the auditory canal.

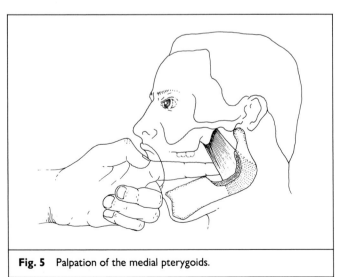

Fig. 5   Palpation of the medial pterygoids.

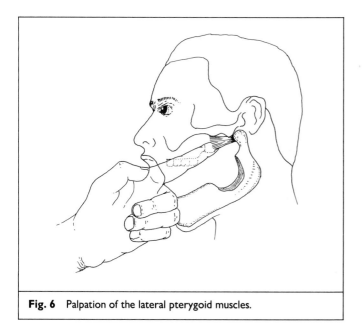

Fig. 6   Palpation of the lateral pterygoid muscles.

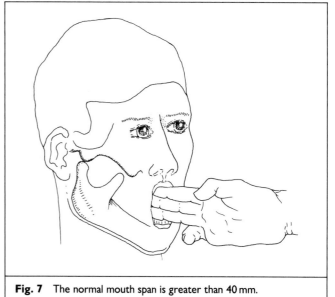

Fig. 7   The normal mouth span is greater than 40 mm.

gently against resistance and then to move the jaw laterally. This muscle has clinical importance, for if it is traumatised secondary to a stretch injury, it may go into spasm and cause temporomandibular joint pain, as well as asymmetrical sideways motion of the jaw.

To examine temporalis, palpate over the temporal area with the jaw relaxed and clenched. Remember that the muscle covers a wide area over the temple. The patient may well locate the area of tenderness.

The muscles of the neck and shoulder may also require examination. The ear should be examined auroscopically if indicated.

Range of motion

Normally one can open the mouth wide enough to insert three fingers between the incisor teeth (c. 35–50 mm, normally greater than 40 mm (Fig. 7). Care should be taken to keep the lower jaw protruded during this measurement, because maximal opening of the mandible depends on adequate forward positioning of the lower jaw as well as on the degree of vertical motion. Note any deviation on opening or premature contacts.

The temporomandibular joint also allows the jaw to glide forward or protrude. Normally it can protrude far enough for the bottom teeth to be in front of the upper teeth (usually more than 10 mm).

Lateral motion of the jaw is measured by partially opening the mouth, protruding the lower jaw, and then moving the lower jaw from side to side. Movement should be equal and in the region of 10 mm. It is best to evaluate lateral motion (normally 1–2 cm) with the jaw protruded as far as possible, as the position of the mandible in the anteroposterior

direction can cause considerable variation in the degree of lateral motion of the jaw. Lateral movement is lost earlier and to a greater degree than vertical movement.

Limited opening or deviated mandibular movements are frequently seen on examination but patients are themselves often only aware of the limitation of opening. The temporomandibular pain syndrome is more often seen unilaterally, and the associated unilateral muscle spasm results in deviation of the mandible to the affected side. Deviation is clearly seen when the mouth is opened and viewed from the front.

Muscle and neurological examination

The muscles that close the mandible are the temporalis (deep temporal branches of the mandibular division of the facial nerve, C7), the masseter (masseteric nerve from the mandibular division of trigeminal nerve, C5) and the medial pterygoid (medial pterygoid nerve of the mandibular division of the trigeminal nerve). These muscles may be tested by forcing the closed mouth into an open position, and the size, firmness and strength of the temporalis and masseter muscles can be determined by palpation.

The muscles that open the mouth are the lateral pterygoid and the suprahyoid muscles. These consist of the digastric (mandibular division of the trigeminal nerve to the posterior belly and the facial nerve to the anterior belly), the mylohyoid (mandibular division of the trigeminal nerve), and the geniohyoid (hypoglossal nerve, C1). To test the muscles that open the mouth ask the patient to open against a resisting hand under the jaw. Normally he can open his mouth

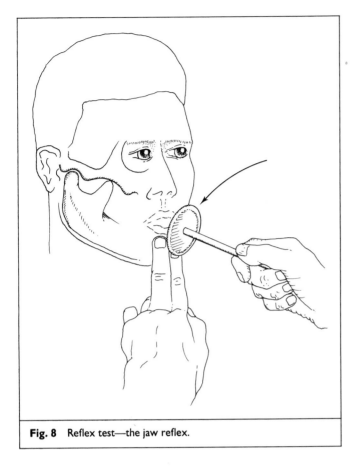

Fig. 8   Reflex test—the jaw reflex.

movement but independent of local oral or dental disease.

It is most commonly seen in young people, being twice as common in women. It is usually a self-limiting condition with a time course of 3–9 months. The majority of patients respond to reassurance, but in 5% the pain is persistent and requires treatment.

Additional Tests

Radiography

Conventional radiographs of the temporomandibular joint may not accurately reflect the joint components and their spatial relationships. These limitations may lead to an under-diagnosis of joint defects.

Tomography is superior as this can reproduce small changes in the central portion of the joint but this does expose the patient to more radiation. Computed tomography scanning and magnetic resonance imaging are increasingly being used.

Arthrography has assumed an important role in the diagnosis of the temporomandibular joint. Defects in the position or structure of the joint, disc and its attachments can be determined, and displacement or perforation of the disc, irregularities in the posterior attachment of the disc, and adhesions can be detected. The most common soft-tissue derangement of the joint has been shown in several studies using arthrography to be anterior disc placement.

Arthroscopy

Arthroscopic examination of the temporomandibular joint is increasingly being carried out. It is best performed under general anaesthesia, but may be performed under local anaesthesia with sedation. Only the upper joint space can be visualised.

Electromyography

One of the major criteria in diagnosing temporomandibular joint dysfunction is to find tenderness to palpation in one or more of the muscles of mastication and increased muscle activity. Electromyography provides an objective means of monitoring changes in muscle activity and is an important component of biofeedback treatment. Auditory or visual electromyographic feedback supplies information to the patient concerning muscle activity.

Injection Treatment

Painful temporomandibular joints often respond to local injection treatment. Symptoms responding

against maximum resistance. To test the pterygoids on the left side ask the patient to move the mandible forward and laterally to the right side against graded resistance, the examiner's hands being placed near the front of the mandible on the right side. Similarly the right side muscles can be tested with the hand on the left side of the mandible.

The *jaw reflex* is a stretch reflex involving the masseter and temporalis muscles. The 5th cranial (trigeminal) nerve innervates these muscles and mediates the reflex arc. Place a finger over the chin with the mouth slightly open; tapping the finger with a tendon hammer will elicit a reflex and close the mouth (Fig. 8).

Teeth and mouth

Note any carious teeth, restorations or dentures present. The attrition of teeth may indicate a grinding habit and a full occlusal analysis may be indicated.

Temporomandibular pain syndrome

This is also known by several other names, such as myofascial pain dysfunction. It can be defined as a chronic or acute musculoskeletal pain or dysfunction of the masticatory system, aggravated by jaw include pain on chewing, inability fully to open the mouth, swelling and local tenderness.

The injection is made with the patient relaxed in the sitting or reclining position, with the head supported. The joint-line can be felt by placing the finger in front of the tragus, and the condyle of the mandible can be felt to move on opening and closing the mouth. The injection is made with a 23-gauge needle using 1% lignocaine to anaesthetise the track. The direction of entry is slightly upwards, and the ease of injection is the best guide to ensuring that the needle point is in the joint cavity. Ten milligrams of hydrocortisone or 2.5 mg of triamcinolone hexacetonide is then injected into the joint (Fig. 9).

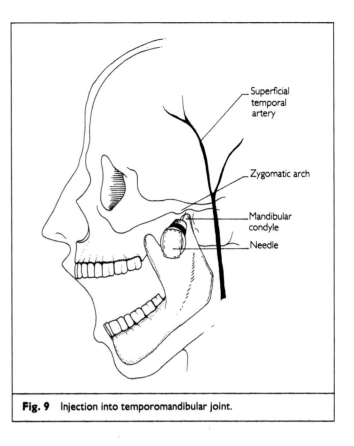

Superficial temporal artery

Zygomatic arch

Mandibular condyle

Needle

Fig. 9 Injection into temporomandibular joint.

9

POSTURE AND GAIT

Posture is the position of the body adopted when standing or sitting. Locomotion is the translation of standing posture into walking. Gait is the description of the manner of walking (or running).

POSTURE

The Evolution of Standing Posture

The length and strength of the lower limbs, the instruments of support and locomotion are very striking and peculiar to humans. They are equal in length to the trunk and head together in normal subjects, but limb length is greater in Marfan's syndrome. Gluteus maximus, rudimentary in many animals, is the largest muscle of the human body, because of its importance in upright stance.

The *feet* are the only surface of support and are the primary agents of locomotion; they are characterised by

- longitudinal and transverse arches to allow efficient transfer of weight and stress;
- rigidity in a closed kinetic chain with strong ligamentous support to provide mechanical advantage and a rigid lever.

Mechanisms of Control of Posture

Structural Locking

The locking mechanism permits standing posture of the lower limbs with little muscular activity once a static position is achieved.

The capsule of the *hip joint* is progressively twisted and shortened as the thigh extends. When full extension is reached, the surfaces are fully congruent and no further extension is possible. The *knee joint* locks in extension, blocking further extension, and can hold a position without muscular action, so long as the weight line for the body above the knee falls in front of the centre of rotation of the joint. The joints of the *hindfoot* (subtalar and midtarsal) lock and unlock simultaneously at heel-strike and forefoot loading, thus providing an efficient rigid lever and shock absorption, respectively.

Muscular activity in posture control

During normal standing, activity is usually found in soleus and gastrocnemius, but consistent activity is usually absent in ankle dorsiflexors, quadriceps and hamstrings.

Under loads of 50–100 kg the passive structures (ligaments, etc.) appear sufficient to control joint position, but over 200 kg the muscles come progressively into play. The first line of defence, therefore, of the arches of the feet is ligamentous, while the muscles form a dynamic reserve called upon reflexly by excessive loads, including the take-off phase in walking.

Stretch reflexes

These can be regarded as a control system that can keep constant the length of a muscle, or rather nearly constant. For a system to become self-balancing, the muscle must be sensitive to the extent of the load and become quiescent when the load falls.

Sensory Function in Posture and Gait

Optimum control of balance, with the effects of gravity, requires continuous monitoring of body position. Control of posture and gait in man involves the activation of preprogrammed patterns of muscle activity which are initiated and modulated by complex control pathways. These carry information from the eyes, the labyrinths and somatosensory sources, providing details of the postural effects of muscle activity. In a healthy individual these sensory inputs provide more information than is normally necessary, so that it is not critical if information from one sensory source is lost, for example by eye closure.

Physiological Sensory Imbalance

This can be demonstrated in the normal subject by removing one sensory input (eye closure) and then reducing the reliability of information from other sources (attempt to balance on one foot with the head fully extended, a position in which the vestibular apparatus no longer functions optimally). This head extension vertigo (Brandt, 1981) is an example of physiological imbalance. The experience of vertigo is linked to impaired perception of a stationary environment. Although lack of one sensory channel rarely manifests as clinically significant instability in everyday life, the demands of balancing tasks in some sports do mean that such a deficit may declare itself by instability during competition. If the history suggests this, it is important to recreate the conditions in which it is encountered.

Examination

A careful check should be made of the posture adopted in the normal standing position and in sitting. Examine from in front and then, standing behind the subject, note:

- the position of the head and neck (Fig. 1),
- any difference in the height at which the shoulders are held (Fig. 1),
- the line of the thoracolumbar spine,
- the alignment of the iliac crests (Fig. 1),
- the position of the patellae and alignment of the knee (Fig. 2),
- the position of the feet (pronated or supinated) (Fig. 3).

Assess whether abnormal posture is spinal (*see* Chapter 4) or related to lower limb change.

Examination for lower limb causes of abnormal posture

Leg Length Inequality

This can be assessed with the patient standing, by noting a tilt in a line drawn across from the posterior superior iliac spines (compare Fig. 1 and Fig. 7). Formal measurement is made by tape measure from the anterior superior iliac spine to the medial malleolus of the ankle and comparison made with the opposite side (Fig. 4). Discrepancy confirms *true leg length inequality*.

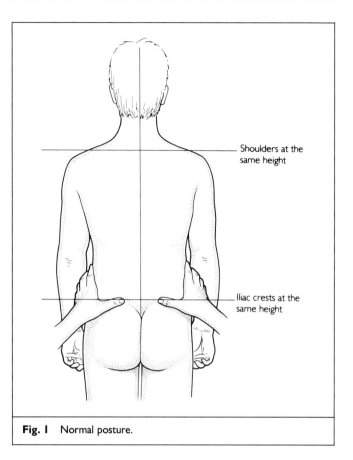

Fig. 1 Normal posture.

Shoulders at the same height

Iliac crests at the same height

The site of the shortening should be determined if possible by direct comparison with the opposite side (Fig. 5). Measurement inequality from umbilicus to medial malleoli indicates *apparent shortening*.

An inequality of about 2 cm or more tends to overload lower limb joints, because of changes in load line. In runners the effects are often amplified and smaller inequalities may become important.

Miserable malalignment syndrome

In this syndrome there is internal rotation of the tibia, the calcaneum everts and the forefoot abducts on the rearfoot as the talus adducts. The medial longitudinal arch is lowered and the foot relatively dorsiflexes, so that the centre of gravity (load line) is medial to the foot: this results in functional valgus at the knee with functional increased Q angle (Fig. 6). Quadriceps contraction pulls the patella laterally.

This syndrome can produce, particularly in runners:

- patellofemoral pain;
- medial tibial pain (shin splints) due to overstressing of the tibialis posterior, as it attempts to counteract excessive pronation;
- stretching of the deltoid ligament and the lateral ligament of the ankle;
- medial plantar fascial stretch;
- abductovalgus deformity of the hallux.

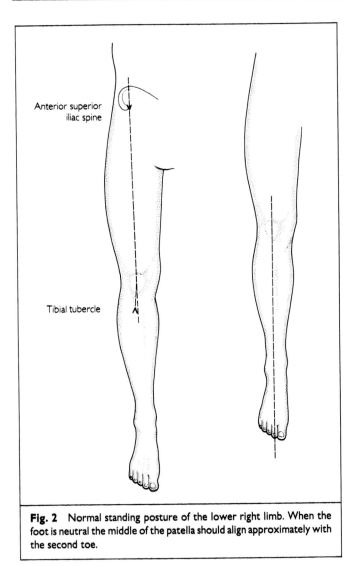

Fig. 2   Normal standing posture of the lower right limb. When the foot is neutral the middle of the patella should align approximately with the second toe.

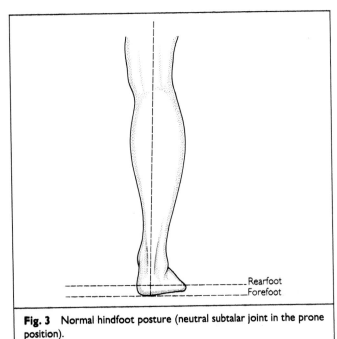

Fig. 3   Normal hindfoot posture (neutral subtalar joint in the prone position).

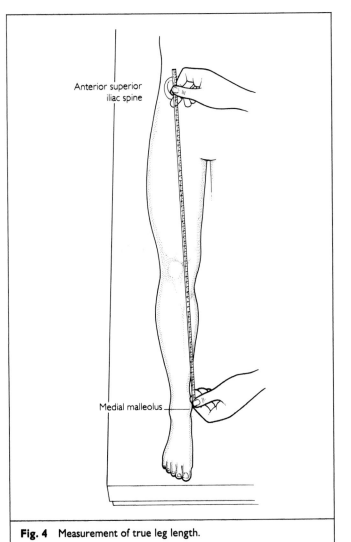

Fig. 4   Measurement of true leg length.

Excessive unilateral foot pronation

Here, calcaneal valgus and functional valgus at the knee are seen (Fig. 7). These result in a *functionally short leg* and a postural scoliosis, correcting on sitting or lying. The right scapula is lower than the left and there is compensation at the cervical region.

The load line

The *load line* in standing is *vertical* from the position of the *centre of mass*. Standing on one foot—if possible—will indicate the position of the load line in relation to lower limb joints. A load line passing to one side of a joint indicates a turning moment being applied to that joint through the body-weight, resulting in potential joint wear and soft-tissue strain. Running, and particularly road-running, will frequently bring out relatively minor loading abnormalities and produce sports injuries of the overuse type. It is vital, therefore, that management involves both short-term treatment of the injury and correction of any imbalance.

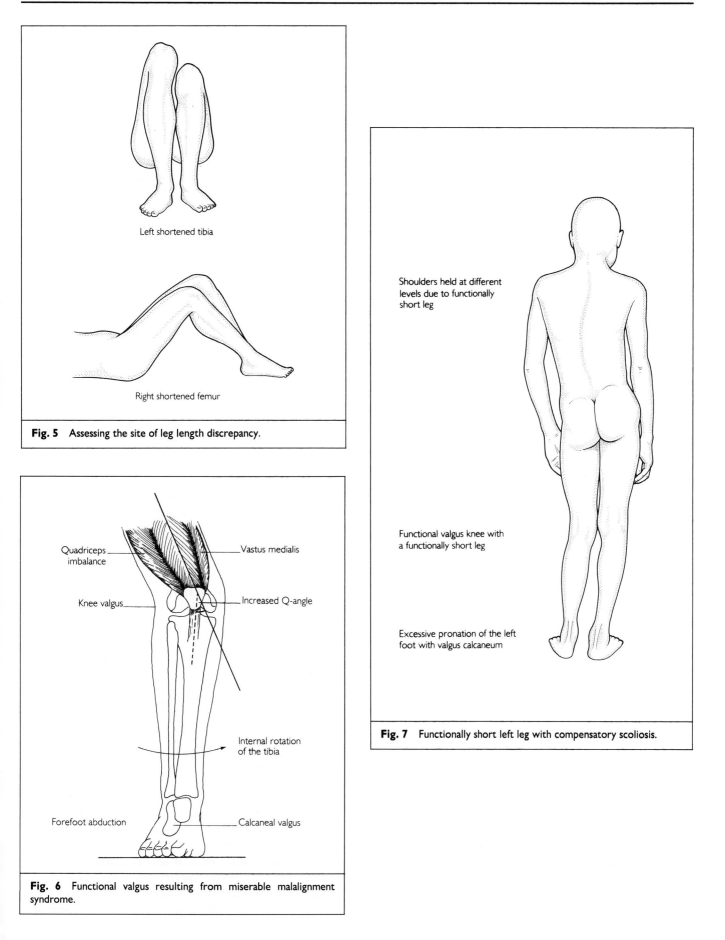

Fig. 5 Assessing the site of leg length discrepancy.

Left shortened tibia

Right shortened femur

Quadriceps imbalance

Vastus medialis

Knee valgus

Increased Q-angle

Internal rotation of the tibia

Forefoot abduction

Calcaneal valgus

Fig. 6 Functional valgus resulting from miserable malalignment syndrome.

Shoulders held at different levels due to functionally short leg

Functional valgus knee with a functionally short leg

Excessive pronation of the left foot with valgus calcaneum

Fig. 7 Functionally short left leg with compensatory scoliosis.

GAIT

Normal gait is a complete co-ordinated sum of the body's movement which results in forward progression of the body in the desired direction. It involves all segments of the body, in weight-bearing, in counterbalancing motion, or in maintaining correct alignment and orientation of the body parts. The integration of all these activities must be co-ordinated and simultaneous, since interference with a single part will result in altered function of the remaining components.

Walking is a process of extraordinary complexity, in which multiple individual motions occur at many sites simultaneously in the three planes of space. In the biomechanics of locomotion there is a long chain of interlinked mechanisms from spine to distal toe. The six major determinants of gait are:

- pelvic rotation,
- pelvic tilt,
- lateral pelvic displacement,
- knee extension and flexion,
- ankle joint dorsiflexion,
- subtalar and midtarsal joint function.

Should there be a fault in the system, since there is a large amount of 'engineering redundancy', compensation usually occurs elsewhere so that the individual's mobility is retained. However, this compensation may later cause mechanical stress, because forces are being transmitted through the wrong anatomical site or may become greater than the design limits: bone and soft tissues increase in strength in response to extra loading, but joint surfaces may be damaged by unusual loading forces.

The human race is more suited to natural surfaces with varying terrain, allowing a variety of foot plant, joint positions and muscle function, hence the use of various functional motor units. We have not evolved adaptions to hard unyielding artificial surfaces, as evidenced by the high injury rate in road runners. This is reflected in the rapid impact spike seen in running on hard surfaces, but not on natural surfaces, which decreases the rate of impact motion.

A brief review of the biomechanics of normal walking is essential to the understanding of abnormal walking patterns.

Gait cycle

The phases of the normal gait cycle are illustrated in Fig. 8 and comprise:

- heel contact,
- forefoot contact,
- heel-off,
- toe-off.

The components of these phases illustrated in Fig. 9 can be summarised as follows:

Heel contact phase/forefoot contact phase: *the tibialis anterior* dorsiflexes the ankle and inverts the foot and so prevents the sudden slap of excess plantar flexion: it also supinates the forefoot with initial lateral heel contact. The forefoot loads from lateral to medial as the tibialis anterior relaxes and the forefoot everts. There is deceleration of rearfoot pronation by *tibialis posterior* which also reduces internal rotation of the leg when the forefoot touches the ground. *Flexor digitorum longus* and *gastrocnemii* (which also maintain knee flexion) complete subtalar deceleration.

Midstance: There is deceleration of anterior momentum of the leg and knee extension (*gastrocnemii* simultaneously tenses preventing knee hyperextension). There is acceleration of subtalar, supination and tibial external rotation. Linear acceleration of the trunk carries the femur and tibia forward over the foot, so the ankle dorsiflexes and heel lifts.

There is stabilisation of the lesser tarsus, metatarsus and rays 2, 3 and 4 and stabilisation of 1st ray metatarsus and cuneiform) and 5th metatarsus.

Propulsive phase: With heel-lift, the ankle joint plantar flexes. There is transverse stabilisation of the metatarsal heads and medial transfer of body weight. Propulsion occurs through the lesser digits acting as a rigid beam and the hallux with sesamoid sliding function.

Swing phase: Following toe-off (forefront clearance) the ankle and 1st ray dorsiflex, the forefoot supinates at metatarsus and there is rearfoot pronation at the subtalar joint. Heel contact occurs at the end of the swing phase and the next cycle starts.

Examination

It is best to assess gait with the legs and feet fully exposed. Ask the patient to walk away from you, to turn at an agreed point and then to walk back towards you.

If the gait is abnormal, it must be analysed more fully to define whether due to a lower limb problem or neurological disorder. Intoxication, hysteria or malingering may occasionally cause difficulty in diagnosis.

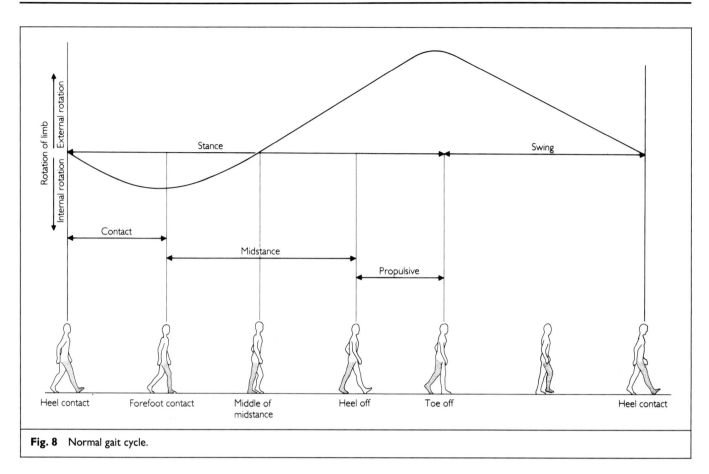

Fig. 8 Normal gait cycle.

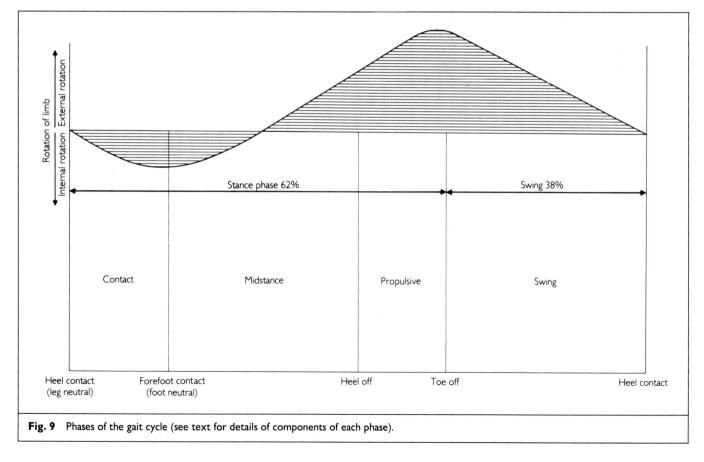

Fig. 9 Phases of the gait cycle (see text for details of components of each phase).

Simple causes, such as a painful corn or osteoarthritis will be confirmed by full examination of the lower limbs.

Since an altered gait due to pain will often lead to unusual stresses being placed on soft tissues, the patient will often present with this secondary pain. It is vital therefore that the clinician uncovers the original mechanical problem. Adequate evaluation of an athlete presenting with pain should therefore ideally include a treadmill assessment of running pattern. Equally, a patient with rheumatoid arthritis needs careful assessment of walking pattern to evaluate the contribution of mechanical factors complicating either established joint deformity or altered gait due to pain. Suitable orthotics may considerably improve locomotion, but inappropriate prescription may worsen symptoms. It is the clinician's role to evaluate which patients merit referral.

Neurological patterns of gait disturbance

Neurological causes should be diagnosed on the basis of the following well-recognised abnormal patterns, and confirmed by a full neurological examination.

A *narrow-based, dragging gait* is typical of *spasticity*. The patient has difficulty bending the knees, dragging the feet along as if glued to the floor. On a hard surface this can be heard as well as seen. The foot is raised from the ground by the patient tilting the pelvis and swinging the lower limb forward in an arc of circumduction, with the toes scraping along the floor. This is unilateral in the hemiplegic gait, the asymmetry making the pelvic tilt and circumduction swing of the affected leg more striking.

A *'scissor-like' gait* is seen when there is adduction and internal rotation of the hips with an equinus of the feet and flexion at the knee.

A *wide-based stamping gait* is typical of *sensory ataxia* and best seen in tabes dorsalis. The patient raises the foot suddenly and usually high, then jerks the foot forward before bringing it to the ground again with a stamp. The eyes are usually fixed to the ground to help compensate for the loss of position sense. With the eyes closed the patient will stumble or fall and often notices the problem for the first time in the dark or on stairs.

A *wide-based staggering or 'reeling' gait* is seen in *cerebellar ataxia*. The feet are wide apart and are planted irregularly, with the arms often flung out to improve balance. There may also be associated titubation, a rhythmical shaking movement of body and head. The ataxia is the same with the eyes opened or closed.

A *stooping, festinant gait* is characteristic of *Parkinson's disease*. The posture is stooped due to a flexion dystonia, and the arms do not swing, often being flexed against the body. There is a slowness in starting, but after small, shuffling steps there is a tendency to break into a tottering (festinant) run. In some patients, if suddenly pulled from behind, they begin to walk backwards and find it difficult to stop (retropulsion).

A *rapid, short-stepped gait (marche à petits pas)* with a tapping quality is seen in deep cerebral corticospinal lesions.

The combination of an ataxic gait and weakness, for example in *sub-acute combined degeneration of the cord*, may result in an increasingly irregular gait with a tendency for the knees to give way suddenly.

The involuntary movements of chorea or dystonia are usually increased on walking and unusual responses may occur when the feet are planted, for example an *avoiding response*, when the toes extend away from the floor or the *grasping response* when the feet appear stuck to the floor.

A *waddling gait*, like a duck, is due to the problem of maintaining truncal and pelvic posture, caused by *proximal muscle weakness*, in proximal myopathies, including polymyositis and osteomalacia, and muscular dystrophies. The body tends to be tilted backwards with increased lumbar lordosis and the body sways from side to side, due to the gluteal muscle weakness, as each step is taken. A similar gait can be seen in bilateral hip joint disease with secondary muscle weakness (*Trendelenburg gait*).

A *high-stepping gait*, with a slap of the foot in the contact phase, because ankle plantar flexion is unrestrained, is seen in weakness of tibialis anterior (foot drop).

Typical Gaits of Mechanical Disorders

Congenital dislocation

1. *Unilateral:* the child lurches to the affected side, because of poor gluteal muscles, shortening of the femoral neck and displacement of the femoral head, as well as lumbar lordosis and abnormal lateral mobility.
2. *Bilateral:* waddling gait ('duck-like' or 'sailor's' gait), inclining to each side on weight-bearing.

Coxa vara

- Waddling gait.
- Stands with leg externally rotated and slightly abducted, pelvis tilted down on the affected side.
- There is usually a slight lumbar scoliosis towards the affected side.
- Buttock atrophied, gluteal fold lower.
- Greater trochanter lower on the affected side.

Infective, inflammatory or degenerative hip disease

Gait is lurching over the involved hip in order to reduce impact on the hip (*antalgic gait*). The child with infective or inflammatory disease tends to adopt a position of hip flexion, abduction or adduction with external rotation. This produces some degree of increased lumbar lordosis.

Club foot: congenital talipes equinovarus

The gait is stumbling, due to lack of elasticity. If unilateral the deformity is usually less severe, but the leg is obviously smaller and less well-developed. Essential signs are:

- plantar flexion of the talus,
- inversion of calcaneum (and other tarsals),
- adduction of the forefoot,
- muscles poorly developed and tendons attenuated,
- plantar muscles contracted, but anterior leg muscles elongated.

Note: the inverted foot position is frequently adopted by normal young infants.

EXAMINATION OF CHILDREN

When assessing the posture of a child, examination must be performed with the child *lying, sitting and standing*. Note any abnormal movements or response to movement. Examine for hyperlaxity of joints and for muscle tone. Note, with the child standing, abnormalities in cervical, thoracic and lumbar spine.

When examining very young children, it is important to screen for developmental delay by comparing the child's achievements with the average for children of the same age. It is therefore important to know the normal *average* milestones of development. Table 1 gives a brief guide in terms of posture and walking.

Table 1. Postural and walking development

Baby bringing head in line with the trunk when pulled from supine to sitting	16 weeks
The head can be held steady and erect	20 weeks
Bounce	28 weeks
Sit alone, leaning forward on hands	28 weeks
Stand steadily, *with* support for short periods	36 weeks
Sit steadily without any spinal kyphosis	40 weeks
Walk *without* support	12 months
Run, stiffly	18 months
Run without falling	24 months

Shortening

On finding true shortening in the child, determine the cause by examining for:

- *Shortness of femur or tibia*, by direct comparison and measurement (*see* Fig. 6): this can be due to fracture or premature epiphyseal closure (consider skeletal dysplasia if bilateral).
- *Soft tissue contractures*, with flexion deformity of hip, knee or ankle.
- *Joint disease of the hip:* congenital dislocation, slipped femoral epiphysis.
- *Knee disorders:* congenital genu valgum or varum.
- *Foot conditions:* congenital metatarsus varus, peroneal spastic foot, club foot deformity (congenital talipes equinovarus).

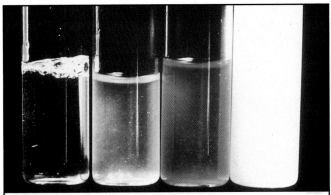

Fig. 1 Macroscopic variation in synovial fluid (SF) colour, turbidity and viscosity: (1) normal, (2) 'inflammatory SF', (3) haemarthrosis, (4) milky SF (cholesterol).

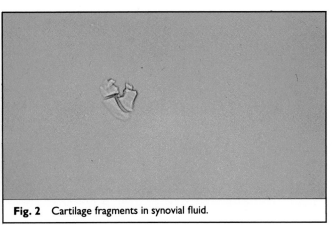

Fig. 2 Cartilage fragments in synovial fluid.

Fig. 3 Diagrammatic representation of a monosodium urate monohydrate crystal viewed down a polarising microscope.

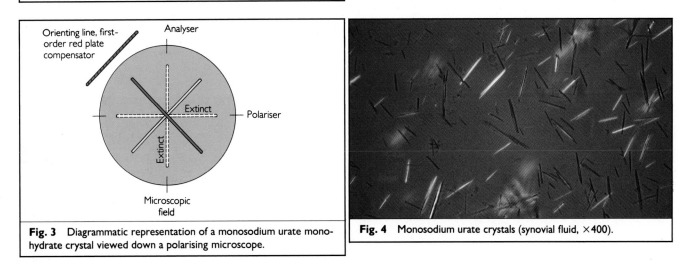

Fig. 4 Monosodium urate crystals (synovial fluid, ×400).

Fig. 5 Tophus aspirate (×400) showing sheets of monosodium urate monohydrate crystals.

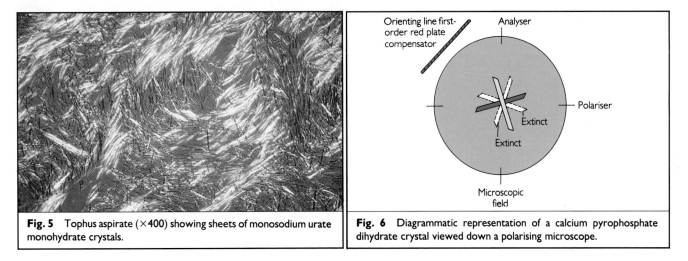

Fig. 6 Diagrammatic representation of a calcium pyrophosphate dihydrate crystal viewed down a polarising microscope.

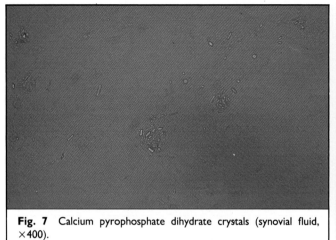

Fig. 7 Calcium pyrophosphate dihydrate crystals (synovial fluid, ×400).

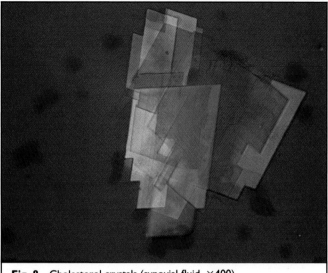

Fig. 8 Cholesterol crystals (synovial fluid, ×400).

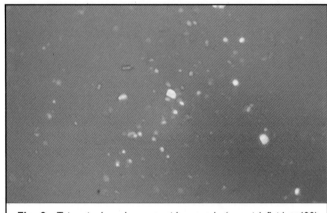

Fig. 9 Triamcinolone hexacetonide crystals (synovial fluid ×400) apparent 1 week after injection.

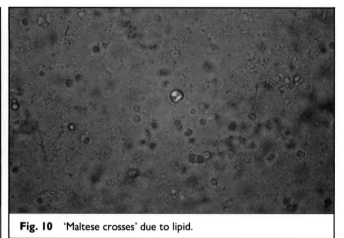

Fig. 10 'Maltese crosses' due to lipid.

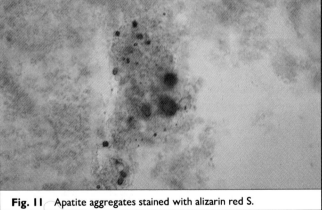

Fig. 11 Apatite aggregates stained with alizarin red S.

ASPIRATION AND INJECTION TECHNIQUES

1

PRINCIPLES OF JOINT ASPIRATION AND STEROID INJECTION

Injection techniques are easily learnt and some knowledge of the easiest routes for each joint is of value to all doctors. Both diagnostic and therapeutic joint aspiration are often necessary in emergencies. Confidence is gained by studying diagrams, watching clinicians and finally by using the techniques.

Aspiration of synovial fluid is essential to confirm diagnosis whenever the cause of the inflamed joint could be due to septic arthritis, crystal synovitis or an haemarthrosis (Table 1). It is also helpful in the differential diagnosis of both inflammatory and non-inflammatory joint disease. Therapeutic aspiration is sometimes necessary to remove blood, pus or large effusions. Pus and blood should always be aspirated; pus inactivates antibodies and leads to joint breakdown, and blood is an irritant and leads to synovitis. Infection usually involves a single joint and usually there is marked inflammation with severe pain, tenderness, erythema and swelling. There may be minimal signs of inflammation in patients receiving corticosteroids or with a debilitating illness. In an infant, there may also be little systemic illness and the child may present with sudden refusal to move a limb.

Injection of substances into synovial joints is most commonly a therapeutic procedure, and a variety of corticosteroid preparations are used. Its local effect in preventing recurrent effusion and pain may be dramatic. Although most peripheral joints can be treated in

this way, this therapy should only be considered when one or possibly two joints are actively inflamed whilst others are controlled by drug treatment. Corticosteroid injections are often helpful in treating inflammatory synovitis, bursitis, nodules and lesions of tendons or at muscle insertions. Occasionally radioisotopes are injected for therapeutic or diagnostic purposes and radioopaque media for diagnosis.

Rheumatoid arthritis is the most common disease for which aspiration and injection is helpful, but it can be given in any condition in which the pain is believed to be the result of inflammation. These include psoriatic arthropathy, ankylosing spondylitis with peripheral arthritis, Reiter's disease and pyrophosphate arthropathy. Injections may also be useful in osteoarthrosis in the acute inflammatory episodes that punctuate the course of the disease, but the use in this condition is more controversial.

The patients who are likely to benefit are those with warm swollen joints, with effusions and stiffness in the mornings. Those less likely to benefit are those with crepitus, instability and severe X-ray changes. The benefit of intra-articular injection is variable, but if it is effective will produce its maximum benefit within a few days. In successful cases, the benefits may last for months, but often it is only for a few days. The first injection is usually the most successful. There is strong anecdotal evidence that the response in small joints is longer lasting than in larger joints.

The major contraindication to intrasynovial steroid administration is the presence of infection, and this procedure should, therefore, never be performed without a definite diagnosis and, if indicated, synovial fluid examination. Stringent aseptic precautions are required to minimise the risk of septic arthritis. Repeated injections may result in joint destruction resembling a neuropathic joint, and for this reason it is often recommended that weight-bearing should be

Table I. Indication for aspiration of a joint

Septic arthritis
Haemarthrosis
Crystal synovitis
Acute large effusion
Effusion interfering with function

Table 2.   Complications of steroid injections

1.   Infection
2.   Pain may be increased in the first day following injection. Microcrystalline steroid deposits may create a crystal synovitis
3.   Skin atrophy at site of injection
4.   Temporary loss of diabetic control in 'brittle' diabetics
5.   Tendon rupture if an intratendinous injection is given
6.   Short-term facial flushing

Table 3.   Indications for injection

INTRA-ARTICULAR
1.   Relief of pain resulting from inflammatory arthritis localised to one or a few joints
2.   Joint synovitis unresponsive to drugs
3.   To aid the correction of deformity

LOCAL
1.   The enthesopathies, e.g. tennis elbow
2.   Compression neuropathies, e.g. carpal tunnel syndrome
3.   Tenosynovitis
4.   Epidural injection of steroid useful in acute lumbar disc prolapse with root compression

reduced immediately after an injection. Complications are listed in Table 2.

Hollander (1951) introduced this therapy over 30 years ago and since then a number of potent steroids have been developed. The purpose is to find a suitable potent preparation with a prolonged effect after injection into joints. It is also important that there are a minimum of local side-effects (e.g. flare-ups, cystic degeneration of bone or bone resorption) and, as the synovial cavity has good absorbitive capacity, a minimum of systemic side effects (Oka and Lähdesmäki, 1980; Armstrong et al., 1981).

Some corticosteroid preparations are crystalline and may induce an acute crystal synovitis if injected into a joint. Long-acting preparations such as methylprednisolone acetate and triamcinolone hexacetonide may prolong the effect of intra-articular injection and are particularly useful in chronic diseases like rheumatoid arthritis.

The indications for intra-articular and local steroids are therefore as summarised in Table 3. The treatment of choice for enthesopathies; i.e. conditions such as tennis elbow in which the inflammatory process is localised to the junction of tendon or ligament and bone. Recurrences are not uncommon but the injection can be repeated.

Procedure

The risk of iatrogenic infection is minimal when a careful aseptic or no-touch technique and disposable syringes and needles are used. Also, single-dose ampoules should be used whenever possible. Sterile towels and gloves and masks are unnecessary. One needs:

-   1% chlorhexidine in spirit or a weak solution of iodine, for skin preparation.
-   A selection of needles and syringes.
-   Specimen bottles for the aspirates.
-   Local anaesthetic (without adrenalin).
-   Steroid for injection: hydrocortisone acetate suspension (20 mg/ml), methylprednisolone acetate (Depo-Medrone) (40 mg/ml), triamcinolone hexacetonide (Lederspan).
-   Forceps for freeing needles jammed into syringes.
-   Gauze and swabs and dressings.
-   A crêpe bandage (if the effusion is large, this is helpful afterwards).
-   Saline can be useful to distend the joint and mimic an effusion if no fluid is obtained.

General points

Careful palpation of bony margins and surfaces before skin preparation increases the likelihood of first-time success, and the site for skin puncture is easily indicated with a thumb-nail mark. In most cases the joint should be approached from its extensor aspect, as vulnerable neurovascular structures usually lie on the flexor aspect. Chlorhexidine in spirit or a weak iodine solution should be applied generously for skin preparation. Towels can be used for prolonged procedures such as arthrography.

To minimise discomfort during or after a corticosteroid injection it often helps to give a 1 or 2% solution of lignocaine without adrenalin first, infiltrating skin and underlying tissues down to and including the pain-sensitive joint capsule. A refrigerant spray can also be used to numb the skin. With skill and practice, rapid insertion of the needle into the joint is possible, in which case local anaesthetic can be mixed with the corticosteroid or may not be required. In some instances local anaesthetic can provide diagnostic information and may also reduce post-injection pain.

The patient

The patient should be relaxed. Tense muscles can make injection impossible, and in most instances it is best if the patient is lying supine with the head comfortably supported on pillows. This also will make it easy to treat a vasovagal attack. Having a nurse present also helps to reassure the patient and is helpful in positioning the limb correctly.

How often to inject

A good general guide is not to inject the same joint more frequently than every 4 months without considering a change in other therapy (e.g. second-line drugs in rheumatoid arthritis. The possible damage caused by frequent injection is thought to be slight, and unsuppressed inflammation is probably more damaging than the possible adverse effects of a local corticosteroid.

Choosing a needle

A 21-gauge (green) needle is sufficient for most aspirations, but a 19-gauge (white) needle may be needed for very large effusions or for fibrinous synovial fluid. A 23-gauge (blue) needle is used for aspiration of the interphalangeal joints and for most injections without aspiration.

Synovial fluid analysis

If there is the possibility of infection, the synovial fluid should be sent for Gram stain, total and differential white blood cell count, bacterial culture and polarised light microscopy for crystals (discussed in Chapter 2, this section).

Precautions

Corticosteroid should not be injected if septic arthritis is a possibility, or if there is sepsis elsewhere. Always attempt aspiration of fluid, and if in doubt of infection do not inject but wait for the result of microscopy and culture. Aspiration of a joint containing a prosthesis should only be done with the knowledge and advice of an orthopaedic surgeon.

When injecting soft-tissue lesions the needle should be jammed well onto the syringe before injecting, as considerable force may be needed.

The patient should be advised that post injection pain may occur and may require analgesia.

The patient should be advised against unreasonable use of the joint for 24 hours after injection. This will depend both on the nature of the lesion and the kind of work the patient does. To minimise time off work, injections can be done just prior to the weekend. Exercise should be avoided during this period.

Dosage

For large joints (e.g. the knee) the usual dose of corticosteroid is 50 mg of hydrocortisone acetate, or 40 mg of methylprednisolone or 20 mg of triamcinolone hexacetonide. For small joints half of these doses will be needed. It is usual to use longer acting steroids for joint injections and hydrocortisone for soft-tissue injections. Longer acting steroids may lead to fat atrophy if used for soft-tissue lesions.

In a large joint, be sure to use an adequate amount of fluid because, particularly in the knee, an injection of corticosteroid alone tends to remain in one place unless diluted.

Follow-up and advice

All patients given an injection should be seen again to make sure that symptoms have improved and no complications have occurred. Advice should include the following:

- The joint may be painful for up to 24 hours after the injection.
- It may take several days for benefit to occur following the injection.
- The injected joint should be rested if possible for 24–48 hours.
- No sport should be contemplated for at least 5 days.
- Supportive splints, such as a forearm band for tennis elbow, may prevent a recurrence of the injury.

Failure to respond

1. The injection may not have penetrated the joint. When training, one can put a small amount of contrast medium in the syringe and X-ray afterwards to check.
2. The main cause of the joint pain was not inflammatory arthritis, but secondary osteoarthritis.

Individual joints

Procedures for individual joints are discussed at the end of each chapter in the previous section.

2

EXAMINATION OF SYNOVIAL FLUID

(Colour plate section for this chapter appears between p. 120 and p. 121)

Examination of synovial or bursal fluid is particularly important in the diagnosis of two treatable conditions, acute sepsis and crystal-associated disease. Synovial fluid (SF) findings may also be of diagnostic significance in a few rare diseases (e.g. amyloid), but for most other conditions SF abnormalities, while often supporting the presumed diagnosis, are non-specific.

For clinical purposes, SF examinations to consider include:

- macroscopic appearance (colour, clarity, viscosity),
- cell count and differential,
- light microscopy,
- polarised microscopy (for crystal identification),
- gram stain and culture,
- special tests in limited situations.

General Aspects of SF Collection and Storage

Although the options for SF analysis are to some extent determined by the *volume* aspirated, even very small amounts may suffice to make a diagnosis. Even if an apparently '*dry tap*' is obtained at aspiration:

- the contents of the needle should still be expelled onto a slide and examined for crystals (unsuspected minute SF drops are often present), or
- if sepsis is strongly suspected, consider injecting the joint with sterile saline and sending the aspirated washings for culture.

For small amounts of SF the usual priorities are a couple of drops onto an alcohol-cleaned, dry microscope slide, the rest being retained for culture. If a larger amount is obtained, it is usual to divide the sample into two sterile plain containers, one for culture and one for crystal identification (added anticoagulants are crystalline and confound crystal analysis). With larger volumes, additional aliquots to consider may include:

- 4 ml into an EDTA tube (e.g. for total and differential leucocyte counts by Coulter counter, or for estimation of complement breakdown products), and

- direct inoculation into blood-culture bottles (for both aerobic and anaerobic organisms).

The volume of aspirated SF can itself be a measure of arthritis severity. Low volumes, however, do not necessarily negate an important intra-articular process: SF may be loculated, and fibrin, rice bodies and other debris may hinder 'aspiration to dryness'.

It is always preferable to examine SF as fresh as possible. Problems that arise if analysis is delayed include:

- a decrease in cell count (due to disruption),
- partial dissolution and decrease in number of readily detectable crystals (calcium pyrophosphate > urate), and
- appearance of post-aspiration artefactual crystals.

Storage at 4°C will retard but not prevent such changes, and ideally SF should be examined within 4 h of aspiration.

Macroscopic Appearance: Colour, Clarity and Viscosity

Normal SF is colourless or pale yellow: it contains few cells ($< 50/\mu l$: mainly mononuclear) and little debris, and therefore appears clear. Its hyaluronic acid content and degree of polymerisation impart high viscosity which can be crudely assessed by allowing SF to drop from the needle tip (normal and 'non-inflammatory' SF both form a 'string' up to 2–5 cm long before separating). Due to the absence of fibrinogen and clotting factors (particularly prothrombin and factors V and VII), normal SF does not clot.

In general, '*non-inflammatory*' SF appears similar to normal SF, whilst '*inflammatory*' SF shows a tendency to:

- decreased viscosity (forming a short string and dropping more like water),
- increased turbidity (due to increased cells, fibrin strands, debris, Fig. 1 (Reproduced courtesy of Dieppe *et al* 1986)),
- deepening colour (yellow/orange/green),
- spontaneous clot formation.

Table 1. Principal causes of haemarthrosis

COMMON
Trauma
Severe inflammatory or destructive arthropathy
(e.g. pyrophosphate arthropathy, rheumatoid arthritis, sepsis)

UNCOMMON
Bleeding disorder
(e.g. haemophilia, anticoagulant therapy, scurvy)
Pigmented villonodular synovitis
Abnormal vessels
(e.g. haemangioma)

Greatly increased viscosity suggests hypothyroidism (or recent steroid injection into that joint).

Blood staining is very common and usually caused by the trauma of the aspiration. If it is uniform, however, causes of true haemarthrosis need to be considered (Table 1). A lipid layer overlying a haemarthrosis suggests intra-articular fracture. Uniformly *milky* white SF may result from plentiful cholesterol or urate crystals.

Rice bodies are small, glistening, white objects (mainly fibrin and collagen) which represent sloughed microinfarcted synovial villi. They are a non-specific finding in severe synovitis (e.g. rheumatoid and tuberculous arthritis). Much smaller, black particles are a rare finding in SF from ochronotic joints (*ground-pepper* sign).

Cell Count and Differential

Cells can be counted using a Coulter counter or cell counting chamber and microsocpe (Wright's stain, or haematoxylin and eosin are suitable for differential counts). Transport in an EDTA tube often facilitates cell counting.

In general, the total count and proportion of polymorphs increase with severity of inflammation, the cell count being one of the features used to classify SF as 'non-inflammatory' (200–2000 cells/µl) or 'inflammatory' (> 2000 cells/µl). The differential is more useful than the total cell count, though both lack specificity and show considerable overlap between conditions. Nevertheless, in general:

- a differential count of > *90% polymorphs* is likely to reflect acute crystal synovitis, acute sepsis, or active rheumatoid;
- a differential count of < *50% polymorphs* is likely to reflect osteoarthritis or mechanical derangement;
- a *marked monocytosis* suggests viral infection (particularly hepatitis B and rubella) or serum sickness.

Conventional Light Microscopy

Occasionally, abnormal cells may be identified, including:

- *polymorphs* ('*ragocytes*') with multiple cytoplasmic inclusions, most commonly seen in but not specific to rheumatoid arthritis, and
- *macrophages* (*Reiter's cells*) containing ingested polymorphs, a non-specific finding first noted in acute Reiter's syndrome.

Apart from cells, frequent findings include *cartilage fragments* (Fig. 2), *fibrin clots*, and unidentifiable *debris*. *Lipid droplets* (which stain red using oil red O) are occasionally seen in severe synovitis (e.g. rheumatoid), and may be particularly abundant in synovial or bursal fluid of patients with pancreatic arthropathy.

Polarised Microscopy

This is the usual method for routine identification of crystalline particles, though more definitive methods are required if confident identification is required (particularly for non-urate crystals). A good quality, dedicated microscope with a rotating stage will greatly facilitate crystal identification, particularly of smaller, less brightly birefringent particles.

A few drops of fresh unspun SF are usually examined, though centrifugation and examination of the deposit increases positive identification (electron microscopy of apparently negative deposits increases positive identification even further). If examination of the slide is going to be delayed, the edges of the cover slip should be sealed (using clear nail-varnish or a commercial sealant) to prevent dehydration and artefactual change. It is very important to use a clean slide and cover slip, and to maintain the microscope as dust-free as possible. There is a marked variation in the 'cleanliness' of slides from different manufacturers, but clean untampered slides are probably ideal. If slides require cleaning, birefringent lens tissue fibres may be introduced; a reasonable compromise is to use alcohol- or acetone-cleaned slides dried in non-turbulent air.

To search for birefringent material it is easiest to scan using a low-power lens with the polarising lenses crossed (i.e. a black background). Once birefringent material is identified, the compensator and a higher powered lens (×400) are used for detailed observation: oil immersion lenses are helpful for small particles. Crystals often associate with fibrin strands and cellular debris, and such areas are worthy of special scrutiny. Crystals tend to have clearly defined edges with straight sides, in contrast to the less well-defined, indistinct forms of many artefacts. Extracellular crystals are often more easily seen, but intracellular crystals should also be sought.

Crystal identification is principally on the basis of:

- size,
- morphology,
- sign of birefringence (positive or negative, according to the convention of the optics of the microscope),
- extinction angle (the angle by which the stage must be rotated for the crystal to alter from maximum to no birefringence).

Monosodium urate monohydrate (MSUM) crystals

These, the most important crystals to identify, are usually needle-shaped (acicular), ranging from 2 to 25 μm in length, and exhibiting strong (negative) birefringence and an extinction angle of 45°. Typical MSUM crystals are easy to identify with confidence (Figs 3 and 4): if any doubt exists uricase digestion of crystals is confirmatory. In synovial and bursal fluids, MSUM crystals are usually numerous and separate (either intra- or extracellular), but aggregated clumps and sheets of crystals are more typical of slides made from tophus aspirates/discharge (Fig. 5).

Calcium pyrophosphate dihydrate (CPPD) crystals

These crystals are variable short, thick, usually rhomboid rods (Figs 6 and 7), 2–10 μm long, showing weak (positive) birefringence and a low extinction angle (c. 15°). With small or cuboid crystals it may be difficult to identify the long axis, and the sign of birefringence may thus appear variable or difficult to determine. Usually, CPPD crystals are present in small numbers, mainly extra- rather than intracellular, and are easily missed. They may demonstrate 'twinning' (appearing as two conjoined crystals) and 'notches' (a chip out of one corner), and they frequently occur enmeshed in fibrin clumps and strands.

Cholesterol crystals

These are large, flat rhombic plates, 5–50 μm diameter, often with a 'folded over' corner, showing strong (mixed positive/negative) birefringence (Fig. 8).

Other crystals and artefacts

Several depot *corticosteroids* are crystalline and may remain detectable in SF for several weeks following injection (Fig. 9). They are variable in shape and size (usually small rods of c. 1–8 μm), show no regular geometric form, and display weak (positive or negative) birefringence. They may occur within or outside cells.

'Maltese crosses' (Fig. 10) are distinctive, brightly birefringent particles that are produced by a variety of compounds (e.g. talc powder from rubber gloves, lipid, calcium oxalate, lithium heparin, dust). *Oxalate* and *lithium heparin* may also appear more rod-like and show positive birefringence. *Brushite* may rarely be seen as large, positively birefringent crystals growing as stars from a central nidus; they most commonly represent post-aspiration artefact. Fibrin strands, intracytoplasmic inclusions, and hairs may all produce birefringence but lack the geometric form of arthropathy associated crystals.

Gram Stain and Culture

Dried smears prepared from a few drops of SF are readily stainable by Gram stain and may quickly confirm the presence of organisms (N.B. a negative result does not exclude sepsis). The Ziehl–Neelsen stain can also be used, though identification of mycobacteria in SF is uncommon and culture and synovial biopsy are usually required for identification.

For culture of most common organisms a fresh SF sample in a sterile plain tube, speedily delivered to the microbiology department, is usually adequate. Inoculation of part of the sample into blood-culture bottles at the time of aspiration may increase the likelihood of ready identification. For suspected fastidious organisms, such as gonococcus, it may be necessary to consider transport in appropriate culture medium, or, preferably, the fluid can be plated immediately on chocolate agar or Thayer–Martin medium and the culture then continued in the laboratory under CO_2. For suspected fungal infections the fluid should be transported in a plain tube and processed for culture on Sabouraud's dextrose agar. Lowenstein's medium is used for mycobacteria. Wherever possible, particularly for potentially unusual organisms, early discussion with the microbiologist (before aspiration) is advised.

Special Tests in Limited Situations

Amyloid deposits in a spun SF deposit can be stained with Congo red, showing up as fibrillar or amorphous material with apple-green birefringence. More definitive confirmation requires examination using electron microscopy.

Apatite particles are too small to be seen by light microscopy, but aggregates can be visualised by staining with the non-specific calcium stain alizarin red S (Fig. 11). At acidic pH (4.5) this stain shows better specificity for apatite than other calcium containing crystals. Such stained aggregates are a common non-specific SF finding, but in apatite-associated destructive arthropathy they are present in large amounts.

Glucose estimation for SF placed immediately into a fluoride tube can be compared with a simultaneous serum sample (preferably fasting since equilibration between blood and SF is slow). In the presence of inflammation (e.g. rheumatoid arthritis) SF glucose falls, but very low levels (< 25%) are highly suggestive of infection. Such simple estimation may be of help in some cases of chronic monoarthritis.

Most other SF investigations (e.g. complement breakdown products, autoantibodies, lactic acid, pH, cartilage matrix components) are primarily for research use, and have little diagnostic significance or benefit in routine analysis.

RECOMMENDED FURTHER READING

Armstrong RD, English J, Gibson T, Chakraborty J and Marks V (1981). Serum methylprednisolone levels following intra-articular injection of methylprednisolone acetate. *Ann Rheum Dis* **40**:571–574.

Brandt T (1981). Sensory function and posture. In: *Posture and Gait Development: Adaptation and Modulation* (Amblar B, Berthoz A and Clarac F, eds), pp. 127–136. Amsterdam: Elsevier Science Publishers.

Cyriax J (1982). Diagnosis of soft tissue lesions. *Textbook of Orthopaedic Medicine*, Vol 1, 8th edn. London: Baillière Tindall.

Department of Health and Social Security (1986). *Morbidity Statistics from General Practice. Third National Study 1981–1982*. London: HMSO.

Dieppe PA, Bacon PA, Bamji AN and Watt I (1986). *Atlas of Clinical Rheumatology*. London: Gower Medical Publishing.

Hollander JL, Brown EM, Jessar RA and Brown CY (1951). Hydrocortisone and cortisone injected into arthritic joints. *JAMA* 147:1629.

Hoppenfeld S (1976). *Physical Examination of the Spine and Extremities*. New York: Appleton-Century-Crofts.

Kelsey JL (1982). *Epidemiology of Musculoskeletal Disorders*, p. 194. New York: Oxford University Press.

Little H (1986). *Rheumatological Physical Examination*. London: Grune and Stratton.

Magee D (1992). *Orthopaedic Physical Assessement*, 2nd edn. Philadelphia: WB Saunders.

Oka M and Lähdesmäki K (1962). Systemic effects of large doses of hydrocortisone acetate and prednisolone acetate administered intra-articularly to patients with rheumatoid arthritis. *Acta Rheum* 8:192.

Owen D (1989). Aspiration and injection of joints. In: *Textbook of Rheumatology* (Kelly WN, Harris ED, Ruddy S and Sledge CB, eds), 3rd edn, Chapter 37. Philadelphia: WB Saunders.

Polley H and Hunder G (1987) *Rheumatologic Interviewing and Physical Examination of the Joints*, 2nd edn. Philadelphia: WB Saunders.

Tubiana R (1984). *Examination of the Hand and Upper Limb*. Philadelphia: WB Saunders.

Wynne-Davies R, Hall CM and Apley AG (1985). *Atlas of Skeletal Dysplasias*. London: Churchill Livingstone.

INDEX